Vitamin D in Childhood

From Biology to Clinical Practice

CHANDRA SEKHAR DEVULAPALLI

Front cover illustration by Prasantha Devulapalli

For permissions, licensing, translations, or other inquiries, please contact the author directly at: **chandev@gmail.com**

Disclaimer: The content of this book is intended for educational, clinical, and research purposes. It is designed to inform pediatric healthcare professionals, researchers, and policymakers. It is not a substitute for individualized medical advice, diagnosis, or treatment. Readers should consult qualified healthcare providers for personal clinical decisions. The author and publisher assume no responsibility for any consequences arising from the application of the information contained herein.

Author's Note: The author's work on this book was conducted independently of his current position at Helgeland Hospital. The views, opinions, and conclusions expressed are solely those of the author and do not represent those of his employer. No financial support was received for the preparation of this work.

First edition, 28 September 2025

Publisher: Chandra Sekhar Devulapalli
Sandnessjøen, Norway
Printed on demand by Lulu Press, Inc.
ISBN: 978-82-694344-2-2

In reverence to Om Tat Sat —
That which is, that which illumines,
that which alone endures.

Contents

Part III – Vitamin D in Pediatric Immune Function and Disease

Preface

The motivation for this book arises from both clinical experience and research conducted over the past two years, exploring the multifaceted role of vitamin D in childhood. While traditionally regarded as a nutrient essential for bone health, it has become increasingly clear that vitamin D influences immune function, metabolic balance, and overall growth in ways extending far beyond skeletal development. Observing persistent deficiency among children—even in regions with abundant sunlight—prompted a deeper examination of the complex interplay between biology, lifestyle, environment, and sociocultural factors.

This monograph integrates my published studies as well as my last one article currently in press, drawing on population-based data, mechanistic insights, and clinical observations. It reflects a journey to synthesize fragmented evidence into a coherent framework to guide clinicians, researchers, and policymakers in understanding and addressing vitamin D deficiency.

All chapters have been carefully crafted to ensure scientific rigor, clinical relevance, and public health applicability. They address ongoing challenges such as defining insufficiency thresholds, optimizing assessment protocols, and tailoring supplementation to individual and population needs. Furthermore, the book engages with global health perspectives, recognizing disparities in vitamin D status and the urgent need for culturally sensitive strategies worldwide.

My aim is to offer readers a perspective that is both scientifically rigorous and clinically relevant, highlighting the broader significance of vitamin D in child health. By bridging research, practice, and public health perspectives, this book lays the foundation for a more nuanced understanding of vitamin D—a foundation that the following introduction builds upon in detail.

Chandra Sekhar Devulapalli
Sandnessjøen, Norway, September 28, 2025

Introduction

Vitamin D has long been regarded as essential for skeletal growth and mineral homeostasis in children. For decades, the prevention of rickets stood as its primary clinical significance, defining vitamin D as little more than a nutrient tied to bone strength. Yet over time, evidence has steadily reshaped this narrow view. What was once seen as a vitamin of limited scope is now recognized as a pivotal regulator of immune function, metabolic balance, and resilience against a wide array of childhood diseases. This broader perspective does not diminish vitamin D's classical role; rather, it situates bone health within a much larger tapestry of pediatric physiology and clinical relevance.

And yet, the research landscape remains fragmented. Studies abound, but they often isolate single aspects — nutrition, sunlight, immune pathways, or select diseases — without unifying them into a framework that speaks directly to child health in all its complexity. Clinicians and researchers are left with a mosaic of evidence, valuable but incomplete. This book seeks to bridge those divides. It aims to integrate the disparate strands of knowledge into a coherent whole, offering a scientific yet practical guide to vitamin D in childhood.

The foundation of this synthesis rests on several interwoven dimensions. One dimension is the perspective of populations. Children growing up in sun-poor northern latitudes, those living in sun-rich yet culturally restrictive settings, and those navigating the health transitions of migration all reveal striking disparities in vitamin D status. These contrasts underscore how environment, ethnicity, and culture combine to shape the biological availability of a seemingly universal nutrient.

Equally important are the determinants rooted in lifestyle. Diet, physical activity, and body composition exert measurable influences on vitamin D metabolism, often tipping the balance toward sufficiency or deficiency. The interplay between adiposity and bioavailability, or between outdoor activity and seasonal exposure, illustrates how vitamin D is deeply entangled with modern patterns of living and health behaviors.

Yet vitamin D is not merely a reflection of diet and sunlight. Increasingly, research points to immune-mediated mechanisms that disrupt its metabolism. Children with chronic inflammation or autoimmune conditions may present with deficiency even when external inputs are sufficient, challenging long-held assumptions about causation. This shift in understanding compels a re-examination of how deficiency is defined, detected, and treated in vulnerable populations.

Disease-specific insights further enrich the picture. Asthma, recurrent respiratory infections, allergic conditions, rickets, and even chronic fatigue have all been linked to vitamin D insufficiency in children. These associations highlight both causative and modulatory roles, suggesting that vitamin D operates not only as a preventive factor but also as a therapeutic adjunct across diverse pediatric conditions.

Finally, clinical translation binds these threads together. At the level of practice, the evidence must be distilled into tools for assessment, supplementation, and public health strategy—tools adaptable to heterogeneous pediatric populations with differing risks and needs. Here, vitamin D becomes not just a subject of research but a driver of decision-making in pediatrics, preventive medicine, and health policy.

This integrated approach is not abstract. It is grounded in the author's own program of research, developed over the past two years across multiple pediatric contexts. Studies published in *Acta Paediatrica* (four articles), *World Journal of Pediatrics* (three articles), *World Journal of Clinical Pediatrics* (two articles), and the *Journal of Pediatric Endocrinology and Metabolism* (one article) form the empirical backbone of this monograph. Collectively, these contributions span diverse topics: the vitamin D status of Norwegian and immigrant children, its links to asthma and respiratory illness, the challenges of deficiency in overweight populations, and its overlooked role in fatigue. By drawing together these strands, this book builds a narrative that is both deeply evidence-based and clinically resonant.

The aim is not merely to catalogue what is known, but to challenge assumptions and expand perspectives. By weaving together molecular biology, population disparities, lifestyle influences, and clinical outcomes, the book argues for a multidimensional understanding of vitamin D in childhood. It calls for moving beyond the reductionist paradigm of "nutrition plus sunlight" toward a framework recognizing the complex, context-dependent role of vitamin D in growth, development, and disease.

Ultimately, *Vitamin D in Childhood: From Biology to Clinical Practice* is written to serve multiple audiences—clinicians seeking guidance, researchers in search of synthesis, and policymakers tasked with protecting child health on a population scale. It is both a reference and a call to action, urging a more nuanced and comprehensive approach to one of pediatrics' most fundamental yet evolving subjects.

In 2025, as childhood lifestyles continue to shift, global migration patterns evolve, and new evidence links vitamin D to immunity, chronic disease, and overall well-being, there has never been a more important time to reconsider its role in pediatric health. This book responds to that moment, synthesizing contemporary research with practical guidance, and providing a framework for clinicians, researchers, and policymakers to address vitamin D deficiency and optimize child health in an increasingly complex world. By bridging evidence, clinical practice, and public health, it seeks to inspire action, inform policy, and catalyze the next generation of research in this vital area.

Selected Publications by the Author

The following peer-reviewed publications form the scientific foundation of this monograph.

1. Devulapalli CS. Vitamin D concentrations were often insufficient among native Norwegian adolescents and children with a non-Western immigrant background. Acta Paediatr. 2024;113(3):411–416. PMID: 38116881. doi:10.1111/apa.17078.

2. Devulapalli CS. Vitamin D intake and status in children and adolescents: Comparing vegetarian, vegan, and omnivorous diets. Acta Paediatr. 2025;114(3):498–504. PMID: 39428613. doi:10.1111/apa.17463.

3. Devulapalli CS. Vitamin D supplements reduce risk of viral upper respiratory infections in children with lower concentrations. Acta Paediatr. 2025;114(5):816–822. PMID: 39727150. doi:10.1111/apa.17567.

4. Devulapalli CS. Physical activity and vitamin D in children: a review of impacts on bone health and fitness. J Pediatr Endocrinol Metab. 2025;38(7):671–678. PMID: 40025874. doi:10.1515/jpem-2024-0527.

5. Devulapalli CS. Vitamin D and asthma in pediatrics: evidence and clinical implications. World J Pediatr.

2025 Aug 31;21(8):760–765. PMID: 40742665. doi:10.1007/s12519-025-00947-x.

6. Devulapalli CS. Immune-mediated vitamin D deficiency in children: beyond nutrition and sunlight. World J Pediatr. 2025;21(9):875-877. PMID: 40880033. doi:10.1007/s12519-025-00966-8.

7. Devulapalli CS. The Global North–South Paradox: Rickets in Sunny Countries. Acta Paediatr. 2025 Sep 15. PMID: 40952060. Epub ahead of print. doi: 10.1111/apa.70305.

8. Devulapalli CS. Vitamin D deficiency and fatigue in children: an overlooked but modifiable factor? World J Pediatr. Published online September 20, 2025. doi:10.1007/s12519-025-00970-y.

9. Devulapalli CS. Uncovering hidden vitamin D deficiency in overweight children. World J Clin Pediatr 2025; 14(4): 110357 doi:/10.5409/wjcp.v14.i4.110357.

10. Devulapalli CS. Modulatory role of vitamin D in atopic dermatitis and allergic rhinitis. World J Clin Pediatr 2025; In press

For a complete and updated list of publications, see ORCID: 0000-0001-5473-9642

.

Part I – Foundations and Determinants of Vitamin D in Childhood

1. Vitamin D in the Growing Child: Metabolism, Regulation, and Biological Functions

Introduction

Vitamin D, a fat-soluble prohormone, plays a pivotal role in multiple physiological processes beyond its classical function in calcium and phosphate metabolism (Prentice et al., 2008; Saggese et al., 2015). Its centrality to growth in early life makes vitamin D not only a biomolecular regulator but also a cornerstone of pediatric preventive care. In children, adequate vitamin D levels are essential for optimal skeletal development, immune system modulation, and overall health (Lee et al., 2013; Bouftas et al., 2024). The significance of vitamin D has therefore expanded from being regarded as a nutrient of basic skeletal relevance to a determinant of multisystem health and a biomarker of pediatric well-being. Understanding its metabolic pathways, biological roles, regulatory mechanisms, and determinants is crucial for ensuring proper growth and long-term well-being (Giustina et al., 2024).

Metabolic Pathways of Vitamin D

Vitamin D can be synthesized endogenously via ultraviolet B (UVB) radiation exposure or obtained through dietary sources and supplementation (Holick, 2007; Clemens et al., 1982). The skin converts 7-dehydrocholesterol to cholecalciferol (vitamin D_3) upon UVB exposure. Cholecalciferol is then hydroxylated in the liver to form 25-

hydroxyvitamin D [25(OH)D], the major circulating form (Christakos et al., 2016). Subsequently, 25(OH)D undergoes renal hydroxylation to form the active metabolite, 1,25-dihydroxyvitamin D [1,25(OH)$_2$D], which binds to the vitamin D receptor (VDR) in target tissues to exert its biological effects (Bouillon et al., 2019; Holick et al., 2010).

Vitamin D Pathway

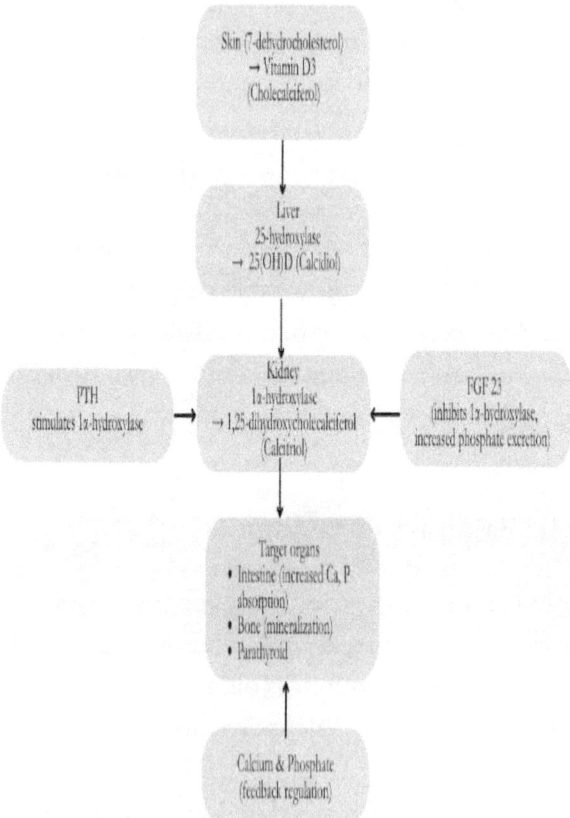

Fibroblast growth factor 23 (FGF23), produced mainly by osteocytes, is a key regulator of phosphate and vitamin D metabolism, lowering renal phosphate reabsorption and suppressing calcitriol synthesis (Bouillon et al., 2019). It plays an important role in childhood rickets and genetic conditions such as hypophosphatemic rickets.

These sequential conversions illustrate a finely tuned metabolic axis, responsive to environmental inputs and intrinsic developmental needs of the growing child. Such mechanistic precision underscores why deviations at any step — whether from sunlight, diet, or enzyme function — can translate into clinically significant deficiencies in children.

Biological Roles in Skeletal Development

Vitamin D facilitates intestinal absorption of calcium and phosphate, critical minerals for bone mineralization. Deficiency in childhood can lead to rickets, characterized by impaired bone mineralization, growth retardation, and skeletal deformities (Saggese et al., 2015; Bouftas et al., 2024). Maintaining adequate vitamin D levels during periods of rapid growth ensures proper bone development and minimizes the risk of skeletal abnormalities. Beyond bone, vitamin D influences muscle strength, coordination, and fracture risk (Holick, 2007). In this way, vitamin D acts as a silent architect of the developing skeleton, ensuring structural resilience that extends into adulthood. From a developmental perspective, even marginal insufficiency during critical growth phases may have compounding effects that extend into peak bone mass attainment in adolescence and early adulthood.

Immune System Modulation

Vitamin D modulates both innate and adaptive immunity (Mailhot et al., 2020). It enhances the activity of monocytes, macrophages, and dendritic cells, and stimulates the production of antimicrobial peptides such as cathelicidins and defensins. Additionally, vitamin D regulates the balance of pro-inflammatory and anti-inflammatory cytokines, impacting susceptibility to autoimmune disorders, allergies, and respiratory infections in children (Jat et al., 2017; Martineau et al., 2017; Camargo et al., 2020). By bridging nutrition and immunology, vitamin D provides a mechanistic foundation for linking nutritional status with infectious disease susceptibility in the pediatric age group.

Regulation of Vitamin D Metabolism

Vitamin D metabolism is tightly regulated to maintain calcium and phosphate homeostasis. Parathyroid hormone (PTH) and fibroblast growth factor 23 (FGF23) are key regulators. Low serum calcium levels stimulate PTH secretion, which activates renal 1α-hydroxylase, increasing production of $1,25(OH)_2D$. Conversely, high levels of $1,25(OH)_2D$ suppress PTH and inhibit 1α-hydroxylase, creating a feedback loop (Holick et al., 2010; Bouillon et al., 2019). Additional regulators include dietary phosphate, magnesium, and endocrine factors influencing VDR expression.

Such immunomodulatory properties underscore why vitamin D has become a focus of interest not only in clinical nutrition but also in pediatric immunology. This illustrates how vitamin D status reflects not only dietary sufficiency but also the complex interplay of hormonal signaling and mineral homeostasis.

Determinants of Vitamin D Status in Children

Multiple factors influence vitamin D status in pediatric populations. Geographic location and sunlight exposure are critical; children living at high latitudes or in urban environments with limited sunlight exposure are at increased risk of insufficiency (Holick, 2007). Dietary intake is also important, with insufficient consumption of fortified foods, fatty fish, or supplements contributing to deficiency (Calvo et al., 2005; Giustina et al., 2024). Skin pigmentation plays a role: higher melanin content reduces UVB-mediated synthesis of vitamin D, requiring higher exposure or supplementation (Clemens et al., 1982). Age and body mass index (BMI) are additional determinants, as infants, adolescents, and children with higher BMI may have altered vitamin D metabolism due to sequestration in adipose tissue (Wortsman et al., 2000). Health conditions such as malabsorption syndromes or chronic kidney disease can impair vitamin D absorption and activation (Christakos et al., 2016; Rahimi et al., 2024).

Taken together, these determinants emphasize the interplay between biology, lifestyle, and environment in shaping pediatric health trajectories. Recognizing these modifiers equips clinicians with a precision-medicine perspective, allowing prevention and intervention strategies to be tailored for specific pediatric subgroups.

Clinical Implications and Recommendations

Monitoring vitamin D status is vital for maintaining skeletal and immune health. The American Academy of Pediatrics recommends a daily intake of 400 IU for infants, children, and adolescents to support growth and immune function (Wagner et al., 2008). Children at higher risk for deficiency—such as those with darker skin pigmentation, higher BMI, or chronic illnesses—require periodic screening and individualized supplementation strategies (Calvo et al., 2005; Giustina et al., 2024). Emerging evidence continues to highlight the extraskeletal benefits of vitamin D in children, particularly its role in modulating innate and adaptive immunity, which may contribute to reduced susceptibility to infections and support overall immune health (Mailhot et al., 2020; Holick et al., 2010). Thus, clinical practice should move beyond a purely skeletal paradigm and embrace vitamin D sufficiency as an integral component of holistic pediatric well-being.

Conclusion

Across these diverse domains—from metabolism to immunity—vitamin D emerges as a unifying thread in childhood well-being.

Vitamin D is integral to skeletal development, immune function, and overall systemic health in children. Understanding its metabolic pathways, regulation, and determinants provides a foundation for ensuring adequate pediatric vitamin D status and promoting lifelong health. As such, addressing vitamin D deficiency transcends simple nutrient replacement; it represents a preventive strategy with profound implications for lifelong growth, immune resilience, and health equity.

References

1. Bouftas F, et al. Vitamin D and pediatric bone health: Important information and considerations for the pediatric orthopaedic surgeon. J Pediatr Soc North Am. 2024.

2. Bouillon R, et al. Skeletal and Extraskeletal Actions of Vitamin D: Current Evidence and Outstanding Questions. Endocr Rev. 2019.

3. Calvo MS, et al. Dietary sources of vitamin D and adequacy of intake in infants, children, and adolescents. Am J Clin Nutr. 2005.

4. Camargo CA, et al. Vitamin D and pediatric health outcomes. Nutrients. 2020.

5. Christakos S, et al. Vitamin D: Metabolism, molecular mechanism of action, and pleiotropic effects. Physiol Rev. 2016.

6. Clemens TL, et al. Increased skin pigment reduces the capacity of skin to synthesize vitamin D3. J Clin Endocrinol Metab. 1982.

7. Giustina A, et al. Consensus Statement on Vitamin D Status Assessment and Supplementation: Whys, Whens, and Hows. Endocr Rev. 2024.

8. Holick MF. Vitamin D deficiency. N Engl J Med. 2007.

9. Holick MF, et al. Vitamin D: extraskeletal health. Endocrinol Metab Clin North Am. 2010.

10. Jat KR, et al. Vitamin D and asthma in children: A systematic review and meta-analysis of observational studies. Lung India. 2017.

11. Lee JY, et al. A review on vitamin D deficiency treatment in pediatric patients. J Pediatr Pharmacol Ther. 2013.

12. Mailhot G, et al. Vitamin D and Immunity in Infants and Children. Nutrients. 2020.

13. Martineau AR, et al. Vitamin D supplementation to prevent acute respiratory tract infections: systematic review and meta-analysis of individual participant data. BMJ. 2017.

14. Prentice A, et al. Vitamin D across the lifecycle: Physiology and biomarkers. Am J Clin Nutr. 2008.

15. Rahimi BA, et al. Prevalence and Risk Factors of Vitamin D Deficiency Among Children. Sci Rep. 2024.

16. Saggese G, et al. Vitamin D in childhood and adolescence: an expert position statement. Eur J Pediatr. 2015.

17. Wagner LW, Greer RG and the Section on Breastfeeding and Committee on Nutrition; Prevention of Rickets and Vitamin D Deficiency in Infants, Children, and Adolescents. Pediatrics November 2008.

18. Wortsman J, et al. Decreased bioavailability of vitamin D in obesity. Am J Clin Nutr. 2000.

2. Childhood Diets and Vitamin D: Comparative Insights Across Vegetarian, Vegan, and Omnivorous Lifestyles

Introduction

Dietary pattern is a major determinant of nutrient intake and status in childhood. As plant-based diets (vegetarian and vegan) have become more common among families worldwide, there is growing interest and concern about the adequacy of nutrient intakes—vitamin D included—during critical periods of growth. This chapter examines current evidence comparing vitamin D intake and serum 25-hydroxyvitamin D [25(OH)D] concentrations across vegetarian, vegan, and omnivorous pediatric populations, highlights nutritional gaps, discusses factors that modify risk, and proposes pragmatic public-health and clinical strategies to ensure sufficiency (Neufingerl, 2023; Desmond, 2021; Devulapalli, 2025). By situating childhood diets within this broader nutritional and epidemiological context, we see how vitamin D serves as a lens onto both biology and culture.

The issue is clinically significant because dietary preferences reflect not only family values and cultural practices, but also biological exposures that can shape health outcomes throughout the lifespan.

Dietary sources of vitamin D and differences by pattern

Natural food sources of vitamin D are limited: oily fish, fish liver oils, egg yolks, and a small number of fortified foods. Because animal-derived foods provide most dietary vitamin D in Western diets, children following vegetarian (may include eggs/dairy) or strict vegan diets are at higher risk of low dietary vitamin D intake unless they consume fortified foods or supplements. Comparative surveys consistently show that vegetarian and especially vegan children typically have lower dietary vitamin D intake than omnivores (Neufingerl, 2023; Desmond, 2021; Weder, 2021). In some contexts, a proportion rely heavily on supplementation to meet recommendations. Practitioners should prioritize individualized assessment for children on plant-based diets, given the heightened risk among vegans and vegetarians in low-fortification contexts (Neufingerl, 2023; Devulapalli, 2025).

This pattern illustrates the broader nutritional challenge that arises when ethical or cultural dietary restrictions intersect with nutrients that are not widely distributed in plant-based foods.

Practical implication: Clinicians should not assume a child on a plant-based diet obtains sufficient vitamin D from food alone—explicit assessment of fortified food use and supplementation is essential.

Table 1: Main Dietary Sources of Vitamin D

Food source	Approx. Vitamin D Content (per 100g)	Note
Fatty fish (salmon, mackerel, sardine)	400–600 IU	Richest natural source
Egg yolk	40–50 IU	Highly variable
Fortified milk (per glass)	100–150 IU	Country-specific
Infant formula (per liter)	400–500 IU	Regulated content

By situating childhood diets within this broader nutritional and epidemiological context, we see how vitamin D serves as a lens onto both biology and culture.

Evidence on serum 25(OH)D concentrations by Dietary group

Population-based studies and systematic reviews comparing serum 25(OH)D between dietary groups report mixed but concerning findings. Several analyses show that vegetarian and vegan children have lower mean 25(OH)D concentrations and higher prevalence of insufficiency than omnivores, particularly where supplementation is uncommon or fortified food use is limited (Hovinen, 2021; Devulapalli, 2025; Sutter, 2021). For example, pooled evidence indicates that when supplementation is absent, vegans are most likely to have lower 25(OH)D, vegetarians intermediate, and omnivores highest concentrations (Alexy, 2023). Conversely, in countries with routine fortification or high supplement use, differences narrow or disappear (Koller, 2023).

These findings stress that dietary pattern acts mainly via exposure to dietary vitamin D and supplement behaviors, rather than being determinative per se. When monitoring vitamin D status, clinicians should interpret 25(OH)D values with regard to season, latitude, and known dietary or supplement practices (Cashman et al., 2024).

These comparative trends remind us that diet shapes biology most profoundly not in isolation, but in interaction with public-health infrastructure and household practices.

This reinforces the principle that diet-related risks must be considered within the ecology of daily life, where supplementation policies, cultural norms, and individual family choices converge.

Modifying factors: Sunlight, Fortification, Supplementation, Skin pigmentation, Adiposity

Dietary pattern is only one determinant of vitamin D status. UVB exposure, season, latitude, skin pigmentation, time spent outdoors, body composition (adiposity), and certain chronic conditions strongly influence how dietary intake translates into circulating 25(OH)D. For instance, obese children often show lower bioavailable 25(OH)D due to volumetric dilution and adipose sequestration, which compounds the risk in plant-based eaters who already have lower dietary intakes (Desmond, 2021). Similarly, immigrant children with darker skin living at northern latitudes frequently show lower 25(OH)D regardless of diet, but dietary pattern can magnify or ameliorate deficiency.

The public-health context matters: nations with mandatory or widespread food fortification and strong supplementation policies see fewer differences across dietary groups (Cashman, 2024a; Cashman, 2024b). Conversely, where fortification is voluntary or limited, the shift toward plant-based diets can increase prevalence of low vitamin D in children.

In this way, the ecological environment—geography, sunlight, policies, and family practices—frames whether the child's plate translates into sufficiency or deficiency.

Understanding these modifiers helps practitioners avoid attributing deficiency to diet alone, instead highlighting the layered interaction between environmental exposures and biological needs.

Clinical and Epidemiological Evidence: Health Outcomes and Confounding

Low 25(OH)D is associated with rickets, impaired bone health, and a range of extra-skeletal outcomes. However, when considering dietary patterns, it is important to account for confounding factors: families adopting plant-based diets often differ in supplement practices, socioeconomic status, and sun exposure, which influence vitamin D status and health outcomes. High-quality studies adjusting for these confounders generally confirm that unsupplemented vegetarian and vegan children are at increased risk of deficiency, but the translation into clinical outcomes depends on severity and context (Bedore, 2025; Carboo, 2024). As such, the real challenge lies in disentangling diet-specific risks from the complex weave of sociocultural and biological determinants that jointly define vitamin D status.

This underscores the methodological importance of robust study design in nutritional epidemiology, particularly when dietary practice aligns with broader lifestyle and socioeconomic variables.

Public-health and clinical recommendations for children on plant-based diets

Screening and assessment: Universal screening is not recommended by most authorities, but targeted assessment is prudent for children on strict vegan diets, those with limited sun exposure, darker skin, obesity, or chronic illness.

Supplementation: For infants and children on vegan or poorly fortified diets, daily vitamin D supplementation is an effective, low-cost preventive strategy. Dose recommendations vary by age and guideline, but ensuring at least the recommended daily intake through a reliable supplement is safer than attempting to achieve adequacy by diet alone in most contexts. The ESPGHAN Nutrition

Committee highlights in its position paper that vegan children are at particular risk of multiple micronutrient deficiencies, and consistent supplementation and monitoring are essential to prevent adverse outcomes (Verduci et al. 2025). Clinicians should recommend vitamin D-containing supplements (cholecalciferol or ergocalciferol as per local guidelines) that are acceptable within a family's dietary ethics (e.g., vegan-labelled supplements where important).

Fortification and policy interventions: Mandatory fortification of staple foods consumed by children is effective in reducing population-level insufficiency. Policymakers should tailor programs to cultural and dietary contexts, while public health messaging should emphasize supplementation for high-risk groups.

Education and monitoring: Parents should be educated on sources of vitamin D, correct supplement dosing, and seasonal adjustments. Monitoring serum 25(OH)D after initiating supplementation is appropriate in at-risk groups.

These recommendations, when aligned with family values and cultural practices, provide a framework that preserves both nutritional adequacy and dietary autonomy.

In this respect, vitamin D policy becomes a model of how evidence-based medicine can respect cultural diversity while safeguarding child health.

Gaps in Knowledge and Research priorities

Comparative data remain limited in quality and geographic scope; many published studies are cross-sectional with small samples and heterogeneous definitions of vegetarian/vegan diets and of vitamin D sufficiency. Prospective cohort studies and randomized interventions that stratify by dietary pattern, supplement adherence, adiposity, skin pigmentation, and UVB exposure are needed to define optimal dosing strategies and to determine whether modest differences in 25(OH)D translate into clinically significant outcomes over the life course. Research must also evaluate culturally appropriate fortification programs and the acceptability of vegan-labelled supplements across different settings. Further studies are urgently needed to inform best practices in fortification, supplementation, and cultural adaptation of policies for plant-based pediatric populations.

Bridging these gaps will require not only rigorous science but also culturally attuned public health strategies that honor diversity while safeguarding child health.

Future progress will depend on integrating both biomedical rigor and anthropological sensitivity, so that strategies truly meet families where they live and practice.

Conclusion

Taken together, the evidence shows that while dietary pattern is a strong determinant, vitamin D sufficiency in children is best understood as a multifactorial outcome where biology, behavior, and policy converge.

Dietary pattern influences vitamin D intake and, in many settings, serum 25(OH)D concentrations in children. Vegetarian and especially vegan children are at elevated risk of low vitamin D intake unless fortified foods or supplements are consistently used. However, vitamin D status ultimately reflects the interaction of diet with sunlight exposure, adiposity, skin pigmentation, and broader public-health policies. Targeted clinical strategies and effective population-level interventions remain central to preventing deficiency.

Addressing this interplay requires a dual view: the microscope of clinical care and the wide-angle lens of public health policy. Balanced together, these approaches can ensure that dietary choices coexist with nutritional security for children worldwide.

References

1. Alexy U, et al. Diet and growth of vegetarian and vegan children. BMJ Nutr Prev Health. 2023.

2. Bedore SR, et al. Consequences of a non-supplemented pediatric vegan diet: nephrolithiasis and nutritional calcipenic rickets. Urol Case Rep. 2025.

3. Cashman KD. Vitamin D fortification of foods—sensory, acceptability, cost, and public acceptance considerations. J Steroid Biochem Mol Biol. 2024.

4. Cashman KD, et al. Strategic food vehicles for vitamin D fortification and effects on vitamin D status: systematic review and meta-analysis of randomized controlled trials. J Steroid Biochem Mol Biol. 2024.

5. Carboo JA, et al. High-dose oral vitamin D supplementation for prevention of infections in children aged 0–59 months: systematic review and meta-analysis. Nutr Rev. 2024.

6. Desmond M, et al. Growth, body composition, and nutritional risk of 5- to 10-year-old children consuming vegetarian, vegan, or omnivore diets. Am J Clin Nutr. 2021.

7. Devulapalli C. Vitamin D intake and status in children and adolescents: comparing vegetarian, vegan, and omnivorous diets. Acta Paediatr. 2025.

8. Hansch L, et al. Dietary patterns among children and adolescents in Germany consuming vegetarian, vegan or omnivore diets: results of the VeChi Youth Study. Eur J Nutr. 2024.

9. Hovinen T, et al. Vegan diet in young children remodels metabolism and challenges the statuses of essential nutrients. EMBO Mol Med. 2021.

10. Koller A, et al. Health aspects of vegan diets among children and adolescents: a systematic review and meta-analyses. Crit Rev Food Sci Nutr. 2024.

11. Neufingerl N, et al. Nutrient intake and status in children and adolescents consuming plant-based diets compared to meat-eaters: a systematic review. Nutrients. 2023.

12. Sutter DO, et al. Nutrient status and growth in vegan children: systematic review. Clin Nutr. 2021.

13. Verduci E, et al. Vegan diet and nutritional status in infants, children and adolescents: A position paper based on a systematic search by the ESPGHAN Nutrition Committee. J Pediatr Gastroenterol Nutr. 2025.

14. Weder S, et al. Intake of micronutrients and fatty acids of vegetarian, vegan, and omnivorous children (1–3 years) in Germany (VeChi Diet Study). Eur J Nutr. 2021.

3. Childhood Vitamin D Status and Population Diversity: Norwegian and Immigrant Perspectives

Introduction

Vitamin D is essential for bone health, immune function, and overall growth. In Norway, a country with limited sunlight during the winter months, maintaining adequate vitamin D levels is crucial. However, disparities exist in vitamin D status among different population groups, influenced by factors such as geographic location, cultural practices, and ethnicity. This chapter explores these disparities, focusing on Norwegian and immigrant children, and discusses the interplay of various factors contributing to vitamin D status in these populations. Key studies by Devulapalli (2024), Kristiansen et al. (2025), and Eggemoen et al. (2013) provide insights into these population-based differences, highlighting patterns of sufficiency among native Norwegian children and deficiency among immigrant groups. The Norwegian experience thus provides a vantage point, where long winters, cultural diversity, and modern health policy intersect to reveal both successes and vulnerabilities in pediatric vitamin D sufficiency.

Framing the discussion in this way illustrates how a single nutrient encapsulates broader questions of public health equity, integration, and cultural diversity in child health outcomes.

Vitamin D Status in Norwegian Children

Most Norwegian children maintain adequate vitamin D levels, largely through supplementation and dietary intake, as reported in studies by Kristiansen et al. (2025) and Itkonen et al. (2021). Despite public health measures, immigrant children, particularly those who are breast-fed and have darker skin, remain at high risk of suboptimal vitamin D levels, necessitating ongoing targeted supplementation programs (Devulapalli, 2024; Madar et al., 2021). Serum 25-hydroxyvitamin D concentrations in infants and toddlers often exceed 50 nmol/L, the threshold for sufficiency, particularly among children receiving fortified foods or vitamin D drops. Seasonal variation remains significant, with winter months posing a higher risk of suboptimal levels, demonstrating the continued importance of public health guidance. These findings highlight how proactive supplementation strategies, combined with cultural dietary traditions, create a protective framework for most native Norwegian children.

This balance illustrates the effectiveness of systematic national strategies, while at the same time highlighting the limits of broad policies when applied to increasingly diverse populations.

Vitamin D Status in Immigrant Children

In contrast, immigrant children in Norway, particularly those from South Asian, Middle Eastern, and Sub-Saharan African backgrounds, have been reported to have lower serum 25(OH)D levels compared to their Norwegian peers. Research by Devulapalli (2024) and Eggemoen et al. (2013) indicates that mean serum 25(OH)D levels in immigrant children in Oslo are substantially lower than in native Norwegian peers. Factors contributing to this deficiency include darker skin pigmentation, cultural clothing limiting sun exposure, and dietary practices with low vitamin D content. These findings are corroborated by studies in other Nordic countries and Europe, which report similar deficiencies among immigrant pediatric populations. Given the multi-factorial determinants of vitamin D status, intervention strategies must integrate supplementation with culturally appropriate education on sun exposure and dietary habits (Kristiansen et al., 2025; Eggemoen et al., 2013). Such patterns point to a pressing need for interventions that do more than prescribe supplementation—they must also respect cultural identities while addressing biological realities. Without this cultural sensitivity, otherwise well-designed health strategies risk low adherence and ineffective outcomes.

Comparative Global Insights

Disparities in vitamin D status among children are not unique to Norway. In urban India, Thacher (2023) reports that up to 80% of children aged 1–5 years are deficient, primarily due to limited sun exposure and inadequate dietary intake. Studies in China similarly demonstrate that 60% of children aged 6–12 years have insufficient vitamin D, with urban lifestyles and dietary habits as key determinants (Wang et al., 2017). In the

Middle East, high prevalence of vitamin D deficiency is reported among children in Saudi Arabia and Iran, where cultural clothing and indoor lifestyles contribute to low levels (Mansour et al., 2012; Ebrahimi et al., 2014). North American studies indicate that Hispanic and immigrant children in the US and Canada are also at increased risk, reflecting the interplay of ethnicity, latitude, and diet (Ginde et al., 2009; Mithal et al., 2009). Global comparisons highlight that vitamin D deficiency in immigrant pediatric populations is a widespread issue, reinforcing the need for international collaboration on effective prevention and treatment strategies.

Placed within this global landscape, the Norwegian case reflects a shared challenge: translating scientific knowledge into culturally attentive, geographically appropriate, and family-centered prevention strategies.

The recurring paradox is that children living in both sun-rich and sun-poor regions can be deficient, which emphasizes that vitamin D deficiency is less about sunlight availability and more about structural and behavioral determinants of exposure and intake.

Key Determinants of Vitamin D Status

Vitamin D levels in children are shaped by a combination of factors. Geographic location and latitude determine UVB exposure, affecting cutaneous synthesis (Holick, 2007; Holick, 2004). Dietary intake from fatty fish, fortified dairy, and eggs contributes substantially to total vitamin D status (Calvo et al., 2005), while supplementation provides a reliable means to prevent deficiency, particularly in high-risk groups. Cultural practices, including clothing and time spent outdoors, influence sun exposure, and skin pigmentation further modulates endogenous vitamin D production (Clemens et al., 1982). Recognizing these determinants allows clinicians and public health professionals to identify vulnerable populations and tailor interventions effectively. Understanding these intersecting determinants enables a shift from generalized guidelines to more nuanced, equity-focused strategies specifically tailored to at-risk groups.

This determinant-based framework highlights that pediatric vitamin D status is ultimately a mirror of broader environmental and cultural systems rather than an isolated nutritional phenomenon.

Public Health Implications

Disparities in vitamin D status have direct implications for skeletal health, immune function, and the risk of chronic disease. Immigrant children are particularly vulnerable, and addressing these gaps requires targeted strategies, including routine supplementation, fortification programs, education on dietary sources, and safe sun exposure guidance. Policies must account for cultural and ethnic differences to ensure equitable health outcomes. In this sense, vitamin D becomes not only a nutrient of concern but also a marker of how societies manage diversity, equity, and cultural adaptation in health policy.

Considering vitamin D through this societal lens makes clear that improving child health outcomes requires both biomedical solutions and inclusive public health systems that respond to population diversity.

Conclusion

Woven through the findings is a central message: vitamin D sufficiency, though rooted in biology, mirrors the broader interplay between migration, adaptation, and public health systems.

Vitamin D status in children reflects a complex interplay of environmental, cultural, dietary, and ethnic factors. While most native Norwegian children achieve sufficient levels, immigrant populations remain at high risk of deficiency. Understanding these disparities is essential for developing effective public health strategies and clinical guidance to support optimal growth and development for all children. Ultimately, the Norwegian context demonstrates both the possibilities of effective supplementation policy and the challenges of ensuring equity across increasingly diverse populations.

References

1. Calvo MS, et al. Dietary sources of vitamin D in children. Am J Clin Nutr. 2005.

2. Clemens TL, et al. Skin pigmentation and vitamin D synthesis. J Clin Endocrinol Metab. 1982.

3. Devulapalli CS. Vitamin D concentrations in native Norwegian vs immigrant children. Acta Paediatr. 2024.

4. Ebrahimi M, et al. Prevalence of vitamin D deficiency among Iranian adolescents. J Pediatr Endocrinol Metab. 2014.

5. Eggemoen AR, et al. Vitamin D in immigrants from Africa and Asia. BMJ Open. 2013.

6. Ginde AA, et al. Demographic differences in vitamin D in US children. Arch Intern Med. 2009.

7. Holick MF. Sunlight and vitamin D for children. J Pediatr. 2004.

8. Holick MF. Vitamin D deficiency. N Engl J Med. 2007.

9. Holick MF, et al. Clinical guidelines for vitamin D in pediatric populations. J Clin Endocrinol Metab. 2011.

10. Itkonen ST, et al. Vitamin D status and policies in Nordic countries. Scand J Public Health. 2021.

11. Kristiansen AL, et al. Vitamin D status in Norwegian children and associations between child vitamin D status, dietary factors, and maternal vitamin D status. Food Nutr Res. 2025.

12. Lips P et al. Vitamin D deficiency in immigrants. Bone Reports 9, 2018.

13. Madar AA, et al. Vitamin D in immigrants in Norway. Fortune J Nutr Food Sci. 2021.

14. Mansour MM, et al. Vitamin D deficiency in children living in Jeddah, Saudi Arabia. Indian J Endocrinol Metab. 2012.

15. Mithal A, et al. Global vitamin D status and determinants of hypovitaminosis D. Osteoporos Int. 2009.

16. Thacher TD. The Burden of Vitamin D Deficiency in Indian Children: The Time is Right for Vitamin D Food Fortification. Indian Pediatr. 2023.

17. van Schoor NM, et al. Public health strategies for vitamin D in children. Osteoporos Int. 2011.

18. Wang S, et al. Nutrient Status of Vitamin D among Chinese Children. Nutrients. 2017.

4. Beyond Diet and Sunlight: Sociocultural, Environmental, and Genetic Determinants of Childhood Vitamin D Status

Introduction

Vitamin D in childhood is often framed as a simple balance between dietary intake and ultraviolet-B (UVB) exposure. Yet in clinical practice, two children with similar diets and sun exposure can present with markedly different 25-hydroxyvitamin D [25(OH)D] concentrations. This apparent paradox reflects a wider web of influences—family routines and cultural norms that shape when and how children are outdoors; urban design and air quality that determine whether UVB reaches the skin; and inherited differences in cutaneous synthesis, hepatic and renal activation, transport, and cellular signaling. Appreciating these interacting layers is essential for designing interventions that work for real families living in real contexts, rather than idealized averages. This chapter synthesizes the most pertinent sociocultural, environmental, and genetic determinants of vitamin D status in children, emphasizing where evidence is strongest and how these determinants can compound—or buffer—risk (van Schoor & Lips, 2011; Enlund-Cerullo et al., 2019; Powe et al., 2013; Manousaki et al., 2020; Revez et al., 2020; Kämpe et al., 2019; Young et al., 2019).

By reframing vitamin D through this wider lens, we see not a single nutrient pathway but an ecology of influences, where

biology, family life, and urban design converge in shaping child health.
This multidimensional framing elevates vitamin D from a biochemical micronutrient to a marker of how social structures, physical environments, and genetic variation interlink in pediatric health.

Sociocultural and Behavioral Contexts

Children's vitamin D status is powerfully patterned by social routines around outdoor time. Across temperate latitudes, 25(OH)D typically rises with longer daylight and declines in winter, even when diet remains stable, reflecting the dominant contribution of cutaneous synthesis where UVB is available (van Schoor & Lips, 2011). However, the amplitude of this seasonal swing depends on how families structure time: school schedules, after-school activities, organized sports, and screen-time habits all shift the balance between indoor and outdoor hours. Urbanization adds another layer: high-rise housing, limited access to safe green space, and heavy traffic can reduce both opportunity and motivation for outdoor play. In many cities, parents' reasonable safety concerns and academic demands further compress children's daylight exposure during the school week.

Cultural clothing practices also matter, particularly for older children and adolescents. In settings where more concealing garments are commonly worn outdoors, cutaneous UVB exposure can be substantially reduced. Importantly, this is not a question of individual choice versus biology but an expected physiological outcome of fabric coverage: less UVB reaches 7-dehydrocholesterol in the skin, so less previtamin D3 is generated from comparable time outside. Where such dress norms are widespread, population strategies (routine supplementation and/or well-chosen fortification vehicles) are more equitable and effective than expecting families to engineer around biology on a case-by-case basis.

School and public-health policies interact with these behaviors. Programs that encourage daily outdoor recess and active transport can meaningfully increase habitual daylight exposure, while sunscreen education—done well—need not compromise vitamin D status. Modern trials in adults suggest that high-SPF, broad-spectrum sunscreen used as recommended can prevent erythema while permitting vitamin D synthesis during typical outdoor activity (Young et al., 2019); although pediatric-specific randomized data are limited, this evidence alleviates a common concern and supports balanced messaging: sun protection to prevent burns, plus routine supplementation for reliable vitamin D sufficiency.

Furthermore, socioeconomic disparities often compound these behavioral factors, with children from lower-income households experiencing reduced outdoor time and limited access to safe play spaces, exacerbating deficiency risks (van Schoor & Lips, 2011).

In this way, children's vitamin D status becomes almost a mirror of daily life itself—reflecting habits of play, rhythms of schooling, and the imprint of cultural identity. Recognizing these sociocultural determinants ensures that interventions move beyond nutrient-centric solutions to embrace lived realities of childhood.

Environmental Determinants: Latitude, Atmosphere, and Air Quality

Latitude and solar geometry set the ceiling for cutaneous vitamin D synthesis. Above mid-latitudes, winter UVB is too weak for meaningful dermal production, so seasonal nadirs are expected even in active children (van Schoor & Lips, 2011). Yet latitude is only the starting point. Atmospheric conditions—ozone, cloud cover, and particularly aerosols—can attenuate ground-level UVB substantially. Urban and industrial air pollution absorbs and scatters UVB; observational studies associate higher particulate burdens with lower population 25(OH)D, including in children (Corrêa, 2015). Families living near high-traffic corridors or in cities with frequent smog episodes can therefore see reduced vitamin D synthesis from the same nominal minutes outdoors. The public-health implication is clear: vitamin D deficiency in polluted urban centers is not simply a behavior problem; it is, in part, an environmental exposure problem. Interventions should therefore pair counseling with structural supports—routine supplementation, food fortification aligned with local diets, and urban policies that improve air quality and safe access to green space.

Built environments also modulate exposure. Window glass blocks UVB, so time spent in sunlit indoor spaces does not contribute to synthesis. Shaded schoolyards, tall-building canyons, and heavy canopy cover can decrease UVB flux at child height, even on sunny days. In practice, this means that recommendations framed as "minutes outside" should be contextualized as "minutes in unshaded daylight when the UV index permits," coupled with skin-cancer–safe strategies and supplementation.

Urban planning that prioritizes green spaces and pollution control can thus be a critical public health intervention, enabling safer and more effective natural vitamin D synthesis opportunities for children (Corrêa, 2015).

Ultimately, the skies above—from clear or clouded light to polluted haze—translate directly into the biochemistry of childhood, reminding us that environment and physiology are inseparable.
Here we see the environment not as background but as an active determinant of biology—turning the quality of air, architecture, and city planning into silent regulators of a child's metabolism.

Skin Pigmentation, Adiposity, and Bioavailability

Physiology translates environment into serum 25(OH)D, and several traits modulate this translation. Melanin competes with 7-dehydrocholesterol for UV photons; darker skin requires longer exposure for equivalent previtamin D3 production under the same UVB dose. In high-latitude settings, this can create disproportionate winter deficits for children with darker pigmentation unless compensated by supplementation and fortification (van Schoor & Lips, 2011). Adiposity exerts another, independent effect. Vitamin D is fat-soluble; higher adipose mass is associated with lower circulating 25(OH)D, likely due to sequestration and volumetric dilution. Pediatric cohorts consistently show lower 25(OH)D in children with overweight/obesity compared with peers, even after accounting for outdoor time—an effect that amplifies seasonal and sociocultural risks (Wortsman 2000).

Transport and bioavailability further complicate the picture. Most circulating vitamin D metabolites are bound to vitamin D–binding protein (DBP) and albumin; only a small free/bioavailable fraction can readily enter cells. Variants in the DBP gene (GC) alter DBP concentration and binding affinity, which can lower total 25(OH)D measurements without necessarily reducing free 25(OH)D to the same extent. Adult data demonstrate ethnic differences in DBP levels and the relationship between total and bioavailable vitamin D (Powe et al., 2013), and pediatric trials indicate that DBP genotype influences the 25(OH)D response to supplementation in infants (Enlund-Cerullo et al., 2019). Clinically, this underscores caution in interpreting total 25(OH)D as a uniform proxy for tissue vitamin D action across diverse populations.

These traits, while intrinsic, do not predetermine health outcomes but highlight the need for public strategies that respect biological diversity while ensuring equal protection against deficiency.
This understanding prevents misinterpretation of laboratory results and elevates the call for context-sensitive diagnostics that reflect child-specific genetics and body composition.

Genetic Architecture: From Synthesis to Signaling

Over the past fifteen years, genome-wide association studies (GWAS) have clarified the core genetic architecture governing serum 25(OH)D. Large consortia consistently implicate variants near DHCR7/NADSYN1 (cholesterol precursor availability in skin), CYP2R1 (hepatic 25-hydroxylation), GC (DBP), and CYP24A1 (catabolism), with additional signals in pathways regulating lipid transport and skin biology (Manousaki et al., 2020; Revez et al., 2020). While many discoveries derive from adult cohorts, pediatric-focused studies show similar biology. In Finnish children aged 24 months, common variants in these loci explained meaningful inter-individual differences in 25(OH)D (Kämpe et al., 2019). In a randomized infant supplementation trial, DBP genotype predicted how strongly 25(OH)D rose in response to oral vitamin D, directly linking genotype to intervention efficacy in early life (Enlund-Cerullo et al., 2019). Neonatal and preterm cohorts also suggest that polymorphisms in VDR and vitamin D–pathway genes can shape early vitamin D status and possibly bone outcomes, although effect sizes are modest and context-dependent.

Genetic effects are not destiny; they set baselines and alter slopes. A child with a DHCR7 or CYP2R1 risk allele may require higher effective inputs (sunlight, supplementation, or fortification) to achieve the same 25(OH)D as a peer without these variants. Conversely, favorable GC variants may mitigate declines during low-UV seasons. For clinicians, the immediate take-home is not to genotype every child, but to recognize that "non-response" to standard supplementation in a minority of children can have a biological basis—meriting adherence checks, dose optimization, and, in selected cases, consideration of bioavailable 25(OH)D or alternative dosing strategies.

These genetic insights pave the way for personalized supplementation approaches, which could optimize outcomes in children with less responsive genotypes (Manousaki et al., 2020; Revez et al., 2020; Enlund-Cerullo et al., 2019).

The genetics of vitamin D illustrates a broader truth in medicine: predisposition informs vulnerability, but thoughtful policy and precise care can still level the field for every child. Thus, the integration of genomics with nutrient policy offers a glimpse into the future of personalized child health interventions.

Interactions and Life-Course Perspectives

Determinants rarely act in isolation. A dark-skinned adolescent living at high latitude, in a polluted neighborhood, who wears more concealing clothing, and has rising adiposity faces cumulative headwinds to maintaining sufficient vitamin D—particularly through late autumn to early spring. Genetics may further tilt the balance, making standard intakes insufficient for that individual. Conversely, supportive environments—regular outdoor school time in spring/summer, clean air, safe green spaces, robust fortification of culturally preferred foods, and routine, affordable supplements—can buffer many biological risks without placing the burden solely on families.

Timing also matters. Infancy and adolescence are periods of rapid growth and bone accrual; deficits during these windows can carry outsized consequences. The infant data showing genotype-dependent responses to supplementation (Enlund-Cerullo et al., 2019) highlight both vulnerability and opportunity: early, reliable dosing can normalize status despite genetic background. In adolescence, when social autonomy expands and family routines diversify, public-health levers (school policies, sports programs, youth-friendly supplement formats) become especially important.

This layered view reveals both risk and resilience, showing us that even when biology, environment, and culture stack challenges, strategic interventions can tip the balance toward sufficiency.
Such a life-course perspective reframes deficiency as neither inevitable nor uniform, but as a preventable imbalance shaped by accumulative exposures that society has the power to modify.

Implications for Practice and Policy

For clinicians, a determinant-aware approach begins with context: ask about outdoor routines, season, skin type, clothing practices, locality (including pollution), and diet—including fortified foods. Recognize that children with higher adiposity often require more aggressive strategies. Use supplementation as the dependable backbone across seasons at higher latitudes, adjusting doses within guideline ranges to hit and maintain targets. In children with unexpectedly low 25(OH)D despite good adherence, consider factors affecting bioavailability (e.g., DBP-related variability); while free 25(OH)D assays are not yet routine, awareness of this biology can temper over-interpretation of modest total 25(OH)D differences.

For policymakers, structural solutions magnify clinical advice: ensure affordable, culturally appropriate vitamin D supplements; modernize fortification policies to match current consumption patterns (e.g., plant-based milks and staple foods for children who avoid dairy); protect daily school-time access to outdoor play; and clean the air children breathe. Because determinants cluster by neighborhood and socioeconomic status, equitable access to these supports is a matter of child health justice, not individual choice.

Embedding social determinants into clinical assessments ensures more equitable and effective management of vitamin D deficiency among diverse pediatric populations (van Schoor & Lips, 2011; Corrêa, 2015).

What emerges is not a story of limitations, but of opportunity—the chance to design supportive environments and policies where no child's biology or birthplace determines their vitamin D fate.
At its core, this argues for moving from reactive clinical management to proactive structural change—a paradigm that situates vitamin D as a barometer for wider health equity efforts.

Conclusion

Seen through this composite lens, vitamin D sufficiency becomes more than a nutritional target; it is a social good, a measure of how effectively societies safeguard the growth of their youngest members.

Vitamin D status in children emerges from a dynamic interplay between daily life, built and natural environments, and inherited biology. Sociocultural routines govern when and how often children meet the sun; atmospheric conditions and urban form modulate how much UVB actually arrives at the skin; pigmentation and adiposity shape the efficiency with which that UVB is translated into circulating 25(OH)D; and genetic variation tunes each step from synthesis to catabolism and transport. The practical message is hopeful: while we cannot change latitude or genotype, we can design policies and clinical strategies that reliably deliver sufficiency across seasons and circumstances—routine supplementation, smart fortification, safe outdoor time, and cleaner air—so that every child has a fair chance to attain the vitamin D levels their growing bodies require.

In sum, vitamin D reflects the convergence of biology and society, reminding us that science informs, but policy and culture ultimately determine, whether children thrive.

References

1. Corrêa, Mde P. Solar ultraviolet radiation: properties, characteristics and amounts observed in Brazil and South America. An Bras Dermatol. 2015.

2. Enlund-Cerullo, M., et al. Genetic Variation of the Vitamin D Binding Protein Affects Vitamin D Status and Response to Supplementation in Infants. J Clin Endocrinol Metab. 2019.

3. Kämpe, A., et al. Genetic variation in GC and CYP2R1 affects 25-hydroxyvitamin D concentration and skeletal parameters: A genome-wide association study in 24-month-old Finnish children. PLoS Genet. 2019.

4. Manousaki, D., et al. Genome-wide Association Study for Vitamin D Levels Reveals 69 Independent Loci. Am J Hum Genet. 2020.

5. Powe, C. E., et al. Vitamin D–Binding Protein and Vitamin D Status of Black and White Americans. N Engl J Med. 2013.

6. Revez, J. A., et al. Genome-Wide Association Study Identifies 143 Loci for 25-Hydroxyvitamin D Concentrations. Nature Communications. 2020.

7. van Schoor, N. M. et al. Worldwide Vitamin D Status. Best Practice & Research Clinical Endocrinology & Metabolism. 2011.

8. Young, A. R., et al. Optimal sunscreen use, during a sun holiday with a very high ultraviolet index, allows vitamin D synthesis without sunburn. Br J Dermatol. 2019.

9. Wortsman J, et al. Decreased bioavailability of vitamin D in obesity. Am J Clin Nutr. 2000.

5. The Global North–South Paradox: Vitamin D Deficiency and Rickets in Sun-Rich Countries

Introduction

Rickets was once considered a disease of cloudy industrial cities in northern Europe, yet today its persistence and re-emergence in many of the world's sunniest regions represents a paradox of modern global child health. Reports from Africa, the Middle East, South Asia, and tropical Latin America consistently show children living in sun-rich environments presenting with clinical, radiographic, and biochemical evidence of rickets and vitamin D deficiency. Far from being a relic of the past, nutritional rickets is now described as a global health problem of both the North and the South, with distinct but overlapping etiologies in different regions (Munns et al., 2012).

This chapter draws upon findings from a recent publication by Devulapalli (2025), which further explore the global paradox of rickets in sun-rich regions.

Sunlight abundance alone does not guarantee adequate vitamin D status. A complex interplay of sociocultural practices, environmental barriers, dietary insufficiencies, and systemic and policy gaps determines whether children in sun-exposed countries are protected—or remain vulnerable—to rickets. Globally, vitamin D deficiency and insufficiency affect a substantial proportion of children, with prevalence rates in some regions exceeding 70–80%, highlighting the scale of the problem beyond individual clinical cases (Cui et al., 2023; Diaz-Thomas et al., 2023).

These data emphasize the critical importance of context-specific interventions addressing cultural practices, air quality, housing conditions, and supplementation access, rather than relying solely on sunlight.
The paradox is therefore less about solar geography and more about the intersection of biology and inequity: sunlight is necessary, but never sufficient, without systems that translate environmental abundance into biological adequacy.

Table 2: Common Risk Factors for Rickets in Children

Region	Primary Risk Factor	Note
Middle East	Sunlight avoidance, veiling, lack of supplementation	Despite high solar exposure
South Asia	Air pollution, dietary insufficiency, crowded housing	High prevalence of deficiency
Sub-Saharan Africa	Low calcium intake (cereal-based diets)	Calcium-deficiency rickets
High-income sunny countries	Migration, dark skin, sun-avoidance for cancer prevention	Often in minority populations

The persistence of rickets under abundant sun reminds us that biology can be eclipsed by culture, environment, and inequity—a condition of global child health not of sunlight lost, but of opportunity missed.

Global Epidemiology: A Paradox in Sunny Regions

In the Middle East and North Africa, case series and hospital data show that rickets remains widely diagnosed in infants and toddlers, particularly among exclusively breastfed children without supplementation and limited outdoor exposure. In Saudi Arabia, large pediatric surveys confirm widespread vitamin D deficiency and associated bone disease in children and adolescents (Al-Hussaini et al., 2022). A multicenter study from Riyadh documented radiographic rickets and low vitamin D levels in preschool children despite year-round high solar radiation (Al Shaikh et al., 2016). These findings are consistent across the Gulf region, where cultural clothing, indoor lifestyles, and lack of routine supplementation create persistent risk.

In South Asia, India and Pakistan provide striking examples. Multi-city surveys in India report vitamin D deficiency in more than 70% of schoolchildren and adolescents, often accompanied by elevated alkaline phosphatase and subtle bone deformities (Khadilkar et al., 2022). A broader systematic review from Pakistan estimated a prevalence of 84% among children and adolescents (Mahar et al., 2024). These studies collectively suggest that vitamin D insufficiency is often silent, preceding overt rickets (Cui et al., 2023), and requiring proactive screening and public health strategies. Urban factors such as air pollution, crowded housing, and sun avoidance during hot seasons compound the dietary insufficiency that characterizes much of South Asia (Ritu & Gupta, 2014).

In Sub-Saharan Africa, the paradox is nuanced. In Nigeria, decades of research demonstrate that many children with active rickets are primarily calcium deficient. Landmark trials showed Nigerian children with radiographic rickets responded dramatically to calcium or calcium plus vitamin D supplementation, whereas vitamin D alone was often insufficient (Thacher et al., 1999; Thacher et al., 2014). These findings highlight that in certain African contexts, low dietary calcium—rather than inadequate sun exposure—is the dominant driver of rickets. By contrast, in Ethiopia, hospital-based studies report vitamin D deficiency rickets in children under five, particularly those confined indoors with poor nutritional status (Lulseged, 1999).

In Southeast Asia, Indonesia illustrates the paradox further. Prospective pediatric studies in Jakarta and Yogyakarta documented biochemical vitamin D deficiency at birth, with significant proportions continuing to show low levels during infancy if supplementation and sun exposure were limited (Oktaria et al., 2020). Hospital series report rachitic bone changes in toddlers, linked to both limited sunlight exposure—related to housing and cultural practices—and poor dietary intake (Pulungan et al., 2021).

Even in Latin America, where sunlight is plentiful, adolescent rickets and hypovitaminosis D are observed. In São Paulo, more than half of schoolchildren and teenagers had serum 25(OH)D concentrations below sufficiency levels (Peters et al., 2009). Similar patterns occur across the continent, indicating a silent public health problem affecting otherwise healthy children.

Finally, in Australia, national surveillance reported an incidence of vitamin D deficiency rickets of 4.9 per 100,000 children per year (Munns et al., 2012). Cases were concentrated among dark-skinned, veiled, and recently migrated families, showing how ethnicity, migration, and cultural factors can override climate protection. Collectively, these examples emphasize that vitamin D deficiency is a global pediatric challenge.

This recurring pattern across continents illustrates that vitamin D status is less a matter of climate than of circumstance—of how societies feed, clothe, house, and protect their youngest members.
When examined globally, rickets in sunny regions becomes not an anomaly of medicine but an indicator of structural neglect—a signal of mismatched health systems, cultural practices, and nutritional support.

Mechanisms Sustaining the Paradox

Persistence of rickets in sunny countries is explained not by lack of sun, but by barriers preventing effective cutaneous vitamin D synthesis or adequate dietary intake. Clothing customs, particularly for girls, drastically reduce skin exposure. Air pollution in megacities, notably in South Asia, blocks ultraviolet B radiation. Rising urbanization confines children indoors, and outdoor play is often avoided in extreme climates.

Dietary deficiencies are equally important. Natural vitamin D sources are scarce, and few sunny countries have consistent fortification programs. In Africa, chronic calcium insufficiency is central, while in South Asia and the Middle East, both vitamin D and calcium are often inadequate. Exclusive breastfeeding without supplementation, in the context of maternal deficiency, predisposes infants to early rickets (Oktaria et al., 2020).

Prevalence data show insufficiency is often more widespread than overt rickets, affecting children across continents and socioeconomic strata. This silent burden underscores the need for population-based preventive strategies alongside clinical vigilance.

The paradox, therefore, dissolves when seen through a wider frame: the barrier is not the strength of the sun, but the filters of daily life that stand between the sun and the child's skin and diet.
This insight emphasizes that tackling rickets requires multidisciplinary solutions—integrating nutrition, environmental health, and maternal-child services—rather than reliance on simplistic messages about sunlight.

Beyond Biology: Sociocultural and Systemic Barriers

Prevention is complicated by social and health-system barriers. Caregivers often lack awareness of supplementation importance, while pediatric services in many low- and middle-income countries do not routinely provide vitamin D drops. In wealthier sunny countries such as Australia or the Gulf states, campaigns to limit sun exposure for skin-cancer prevention have inadvertently increased rickets risk among vulnerable populations (Munns et al., 2012).

Raising caregiver and professional awareness about vitamin D deficiency remains a cornerstone of prevention, particularly in underserved and culturally diverse populations.

Here, the story of rickets shifts from physiology alone to one of inequity, where health systems and social awareness lag behind what science long ago made clear.
This systemic gap reflects a broader theme in global health: that knowledge of simple interventions does not guarantee implementation unless political will, cultural adaptation, and resource allocation are aligned.

Implications for Prevention

The paradox of rickets in sunny regions demonstrates that strategies must be tailored to local etiologies. In South Asia and the Middle East, programs should emphasize vitamin D supplementation, fortification, and safe sun exposure. In Africa, calcium intake must be simultaneously addressed, as shown by Nigerian trials. Across all regions, attention is needed for infants, toddlers, and adolescents.

Global public health initiatives could include fortification, supplementation, school programs, and culturally sensitive sun exposure guidance. Clinicians can use prevalence data to identify high-risk populations, advocate for policies, and implement targeted screening programs.

Coordinated global efforts integrating surveillance, culturally appropriate education, and equitable supplementation programs are essential to eradicate this preventable condition.

Taken together, these strategies represent not simply nutritional policy but an investment in equity—ensuring that no child grows with bent bones for want of a supplement, fortification, or safe sun.

True progress against rickets in sunny countries will come not merely from clinical prescriptions but from embedding vitamin D prevention into the architecture of child health systems, education, and policy.

Conclusion

Viewed globally, rickets is not a paradox but a lesson: that sunlight, though abundant, must be partnered with nutrition, education, and policy if its promise for child health is to be fulfilled.

Rickets in sunny countries remains a paradox only if sunlight is viewed in isolation. Children's bone health is the product of nutrition, culture, environment, and health systems. From Riyadh to New Delhi, Lagos to São Paulo, persistence of rickets reflects not a failure of nature but a failure of prevention. Integrating prevalence and insufficiency data into policy and clinical strategies ensures interventions are evidence-based, targeted, and effective (Diaz-Thomas et al., 2023).

Region-specific strategies combining supplementation, fortification, and social change are required to prevent rickets globally.

Ultimately, conquering the North–South paradox will demand that sunlight, science, and social responsibility converge into coherent action, ensuring that every child can grow free from a disease as preventable as rickets.

References

1. Al-Hussaini A, et al. Vitamin D and iron deficiencies among Saudi children and adolescents: A persistent problem in the 21st century. Saudi J Gastroenterol. 2022.

2. Al Shaikh A, et al. Radiographic rickets and vitamin D deficiency in Saudi preschool children. Pediatrics. 2016.

3. Cui A, et al. Global and regional prevalence of vitamin D deficiency in population-based studies

from 2000 to 2022: A pooled analysis of 7.9 million participants. Front Nutr. 2023.

4. Diaz-Thomas A, et al. Global health disparities in childhood rickets. Endocrinol Metab Clin North Am. 2023.

5. Devulapalli CS. The Global North–South Paradox: Rickets in Sunny Countries. Acta Paediatr. 2025 Sep 15. doi: 10.1111/apa.70305.

6. Khadilkar A, et al. Vitamin D status and determinants in Indian children and adolescents: a multicenter study. Sci Rep. 2022.

7. Lulseged S, et al. Vitamin D deficiency rickets: socio-demographic and clinical risk factors in children seen at a referral hospital in Addis Ababa. East Afr Med J. 1999.

8. Mahar B, et al. Vitamin D deficiency prevalence in Pakistan: common, important, and neglected: a comprehensive meta-analysis. J Diabetol. 2024.

9. Munns CF, et al. Incidence of vitamin D deficiency rickets among Australian children: An Australian Paediatric Surveillance Unit study. Med J Aust. 2012.

10. Oktaria V, et al. Vitamin D deficiency in Indonesian infants at birth and six months: determinants and sun exposure. PLoS One. 2020.

11. Peters BSE, et al. Prevalence of vitamin D insufficiency in Brazilian adolescents. Ann Nutr Metab. 2009.

12. Pulungan A, et al. Vitamin D insufficiency and its contributing factors in primary school-aged children in Indonesia, a sun-rich country. Ann Pediatr Endocrinol Metab. 2021.

13. Ritu G, Gupta A. Vitamin D deficiency in India: prevalence, causalities and interventions in children. Nutrients. 2014.

14. Thacher TD, et al. A comparison of calcium, vitamin D, or both for nutritional rickets in Nigerian children. N Engl J Med. 1999.

15. Thacher TD, et al. Vitamin D treatment in calcium-deficiency rickets: a randomized controlled trial. Arch Dis Child. 2014.

Part II – Lifestyle, Environment, and Body Composition

6. Childhood Physical Activity and Vitamin D Status: Implications for Bone Development and Fitness

Introduction

Physical activity and vitamin D are two critical determinants of musculoskeletal health during childhood and adolescence. Adequate physical activity supports bone modeling and muscle development, while vitamin D regulates calcium–phosphate metabolism and contributes to bone mineralization. Emerging evidence highlights synergistic interactions between these factors, suggesting that optimal skeletal health relies on both regular outdoor activity and sufficient vitamin D status (Devulapalli, 2025; Holick, 2007). Beyond skeletal outcomes, physical activity may also influence vitamin D bioavailability indirectly through effects on body composition, while sunlight exposure during outdoor play promotes endogenous vitamin D synthesis.

Together, these elements remind us that children's bones are not simply built by nutrients or exercise in isolation, but by their dynamic partnership across time and environment.

By considering diet, sunlight, and physical activity together, clinicians and policymakers can more accurately capture the true determinants of musculoskeletal health, moving beyond reductionist models toward integrated child health strategies.

Interactions Between Physical Activity and Vitamin D

Children engaged in regular weight-bearing or load-bearing activity demonstrate higher bone mineral density (BMD) and improved musculoskeletal strength (Specker & Binkley, 2003; Tan et al., 2014). Physical activity often coincides with outdoor exposure, allowing ultraviolet B (UVB)–mediated cutaneous production of vitamin D, the primary source for most children (Holick, 2007). Observational studies indicate that children with higher outdoor activity levels exhibit both higher serum 25(OH)D concentrations and superior musculoskeletal outcomes compared with less active peers (Devulapalli, 2025; Ouyang et al., 2024; Won et al., 2021).

Intervention evidence supports a positive effect of physical activity on vitamin D status and bone outcomes; systematic reviews and meta-analyses of intervention studies corroborate these interactions (see Karimian et al., 2022). In particular, a recent systematic review and meta-analysis found that structured physical activity interventions influence vitamin D–related outcomes and should be considered when designing combined intervention programs (Khan SR et al., 2024).

This synergy highlights the need for integrated interventions promoting both outdoor physical activity and adequate vitamin D intake to maximize bone health benefits early in life.

This dual benefit—stronger bones and healthier vitamin D status—illustrates how daily play under the open sky is both a developmental necessity and a preventive health measure. Such evidence reframes outdoor activity as more than recreation; it becomes a biologically essential behavior that couples movement and micronutrient sufficiency.

Body Composition and Vitamin D

Adiposity modifies vitamin D status by sequestering the fat-soluble vitamin in adipose tissue, reducing its bioavailability (Wortsman et al., 2000; Devulapalli, 2025). Children with higher body mass index (BMI) who are less active may therefore be doubly disadvantaged: lower vitamin D bioavailability and reduced mechanical loading for bone accrual. Intervention studies and reviews suggest that combining physical activity with vitamin D supplementation can improve BMD in overweight and obese children, supporting an integrated approach to musculoskeletal health (Płudowski et al., 2018; Karimian et al., 2022; Khan SR et al., 2024).

Addressing obesity through lifestyle modifications can therefore have dual benefits in improving vitamin D bioavailability and enhancing mechanical stimuli for bone growth. Furthermore, addressing obesity in childhood is thus doubly meaningful: it lightens the biological burden on bone while brightening the pathways by which vitamin D supports growth.

In this way, managing excess adiposity emerges as not simply a metabolic or cardiovascular intervention, but also as an indirect strategy to optimize vitamin D effectiveness in bone accrual and musculoskeletal resilience.

Muscle Function and Neuromuscular Development

Vitamin D contributes to muscle function by promoting protein synthesis and maintaining calcium homeostasis in muscle cells, whereas physical activity enhances neuromuscular coordination and strength (Pfeifer et al., 2002; Devulapalli, 2025). Evidence syntheses indicate that adequate vitamin D status potentiates gains in muscle function during training and may reduce injury risk; this is supported by guideline documents and systematic reviews addressing vitamin D and musculoskeletal outcomes in children (Płudowski et al., 2018; Khan SR et al., 2024).

Ensuring sufficient vitamin D levels may therefore improve performance and recovery in physically active children, further supporting musculoskeletal health. When nutrition and movement align, gains in coordination, strength, and resilience flow not just from muscles themselves, but from the molecular support of vitamin D.

These findings illustrate that vitamin D is not simply permissive for bone and muscle health but actively amplifies adaptation to exercise, underscoring its importance in both athletic and non-athletic children.

Geographic, Seasonal, and Environmental Modifiers

Latitude, season, and outdoor environmental exposure substantially influence the interaction between activity and vitamin D. Children living at higher latitudes or in urban environments with limited sunlight show lower 25(OH)D concentrations, even when physically active (Won et al., 2021; Devulapalli, 2025). Seasonal variation also affects status; winter months often coincide with indoor activity patterns, compounding the risk of deficiency. Public health strategies must consider these contextual factors to optimize both activity promotion and vitamin D sufficiency.

This context underscores that geography and lifestyle can magnify or mute biology, shaping how completely the promise of activity and sunlight translates into sufficiency. Without recognition of these modifiers, interventions risk being overly generalized, while context-sensitive strategies ensure that recommendations for outdoor time and supplementation are both realistic and equitable.

Public Health and Clinical Implications

Integrating physical activity promotion with vitamin D sufficiency strategies has broad implications. Clinicians should encourage daily outdoor activity while assessing dietary intake and supplementation for children at risk of low vitamin D, particularly in higher latitudes or in populations with darker skin (Fatima Bouftas et al., 2024; Al-Othman et al., 2012). School-based and community interventions can simultaneously address sedentary behavior and deficiency risk. Evidence supports targeted supplementation for at-risk children combined with promotion of weight-bearing outdoor activity to maximize skeletal health, reduce fracture risk, and improve overall fitness.

School- and community-based programs that combine nutrition education with structured physical activity opportunities are particularly effective in reaching diverse pediatric populations.

By pairing outdoor movement with reliable supplementation, communities can ensure that fitness, growth, and resilience advance together as foundational rights of childhood. This integration also reframes child health policy: not as separate domains of sport and nutrition policy, but as converging responsibilities to safeguard holistic development.

Conclusion

Seen in concert, physical activity and vitamin D form a symphony of growth—one providing the rhythm of movement, the other the elemental notes of mineral balance and repair.

Physical activity and vitamin D status are tightly interwoven determinants of musculoskeletal health in children. Outdoor activity enhances bone mineral accrual and promotes vitamin D synthesis, while sufficient vitamin D supports musculoskeletal function and amplifies the benefits of exercise. Body composition, geographic, seasonal, and lifestyle factors modulate these interactions. Integrated public health and clinical strategies that simultaneously promote physical activity and vitamin D sufficiency are essential for supporting healthy growth trajectories in pediatric populations.

The evidence thus points toward a unifying paradigm: bone health in childhood is safeguarded not by isolated measures but by interdependent systems of movement, nutrition, and environment working in synchrony.

References

1. Al-Othman A, et al. Effect of physical activity and sun exposure on vitamin D status of Saudi children and adolescents. BMC Pediatr. 2012.

2. Bouftas F, et al. Vitamin D and pediatric bone health: Important information and considerations for the pediatric orthopaedic surgeon. Journal of the Pediatric Orthopaedic Society of North America. 2024.

3. Devulapalli CS. Physical activity and vitamin D in children: a review of impacts on bone health and fitness. J Pediatr Endocrinol Metab. 2025.

4. Holick MF. Vitamin D deficiency. N Engl J Med. 2007.

5. Kamrath C, et al. Sunlight, supplements, and science: vitamin D as a tool for pediatric health care. J Pediatr Endocrinol Metab. 2025.

6. Karimian P, et al. Effects of vitamin D on bone density in healthy children: A systematic review. J Family Med Prim Care. 2022.

7. Khan SR, et al. The effect of physical activity on vitamin D: A systematic review and meta-analysis of intervention studies in humans. Public Health in Practice. 2024.

8. Ouyang S, et al. The relationship between physical activity levels and serum vitamin D levels varies among children and adolescents in different age groups. Front Nutr. 2024.

9. Pfeifer M, et al. Vitamin D and muscle function. Osteoporos Int. 2002.

10. Płudowski P, et al. Vitamin D supplementation guidelines. J Steroid Biochem Mol Biol. 2018.

11. Specker BL, Binkley TL. Randomized trial of physical activity and calcium supplementation on bone mineral content in 3- to 5-year-old children. J Bone Miner Res. 2003.

12. Tan VP, et al. Influence of physical activity on bone strength in children and adolescents: a systematic review and narrative synthesis. J Bone Miner Res. 2014.

13. Won JW, et al. Seasonal Changes in Vitamin D Levels of Healthy Children in Mid-Latitude, Asian Urban Area. Pediatr Gastroenterol Hepatol Nutr. 2021.

14. Wortsman J, et al. Obesity and vitamin D metabolism. Am J Clin Nutr. 2000.

7. Vitamin D Deficiency in Overweight Children: Mechanisms and Management

Introduction

Vitamin D deficiency remains one of the most pervasive nutritional challenges worldwide, with implications for skeletal health, immune regulation, and long-term metabolic outcomes. Among children, overweight and obesity have emerged as important risk factors for low vitamin D status. Traditionally, deficiency was thought to reflect insufficient dietary intake or inadequate exposure to sunlight. However, in children with obesity, the picture is more complex. Emerging evidence demonstrates that vitamin D deficiency in this population is not merely a matter of reduced intake, but a "functional deficiency" driven by altered physiology, metabolic disruptions, and adipose tissue dynamics.

Recent work, including the review by Devulapalli (2025), has emphasized the interplay between adiposity, metabolism, and inflammation in shaping vitamin D status among overweight children. Understanding these mechanisms is critical, as standard supplementation and diagnostic thresholds may fail to adequately address the needs of this vulnerable group.

This shifting understanding moves deficiency out of the simplistic realm of sunlight and diet, situating it instead within the deeper currents of physiology and metabolism.

In this sense, obesity serves as both a cause and a consequence of altered vitamin D biology, creating a feedback loop in which physiology amplifies vulnerability.

Adipose Tissue Sequestration and Bioavailability

One of the most widely recognized explanations for lower circulating 25-hydroxyvitamin D [25(OH)D] concentrations in overweight children is sequestration in adipose tissue. Because vitamin D is fat-soluble, excessive storage in enlarged fat depots reduces its bioavailability for metabolic and endocrine functions (Wortsman et al., 2000; Blum et al., 2008).

In both adults and children, studies demonstrate an inverse relationship between body mass index (BMI) and serum 25(OH)D, even after adjusting for dietary intake and sunlight exposure (Turer et al., 2013; Rajakumar et al., 2011). This suggests that bioavailability is compromised not by inadequate intake but by redistribution and trapping of vitamin D within adipose tissue.

This sequestration effect underscores the importance of considering body composition in vitamin D assessments and tailoring supplementation strategies accordingly.

In practice, the child's own body composition becomes both a reservoir and a barrier, reshaping how nutrients are stored, circulated, and ultimately used.

This highlights why identical supplementation regimens can produce divergent outcomes depending on the degree of adiposity, demanding individualized clinical interpretation.

Altered Metabolism and Inflammatory Signaling

Adiposity does more than sequester vitamin D—it also alters its metabolism. Evidence indicates reduced activity of hepatic 25-hydroxylase in obesity, impairing conversion of vitamin D to its main circulating form, 25(OH)D (Roth et al., 2011).

In addition, inflammatory cytokines released from adipose tissue, including tumor necrosis factor-alpha (TNF-α) and interleukin-6 (IL-6), may interfere with vitamin D receptor signaling and enzymatic activation (Carrelli et al., 2017; Vimaleswaran et al., 2013).

Meta-analyses confirm that vitamin D deficiency is consistently more prevalent in children and adolescents with obesity (Fiamenghi et al., 2021; Corsello et al., 2023). These findings align with the hypothesis that vitamin D metabolism and signaling pathways are impaired in obesity not only by sequestration, but also by inflammatory and enzymatic dysregulation.

Furthermore, chronic inflammation in adipose tissue may not only impair vitamin D metabolism but also exacerbate systemic metabolic dysfunction, creating a vicious cycle.

Thus, inflammation transforms a nutrient problem into a systemic state, where vitamin D deficiency both reflects and reinforces metabolic imbalance.
This dual mechanism—storage and signaling disruption—illustrates how fat tissue operates not passively, but as an active endocrine organ reshaping micronutrient function.

Vitamin D Binding Protein and Hormonal Regulation

Another layer of complexity involves vitamin D–binding protein (DBP), the carrier molecule that transports vitamin D metabolites in circulation. Alterations in DBP concentrations or affinity may reduce the fraction of free, biologically active vitamin D available to tissues. Some studies have observed lower DBP concentrations in obese individuals, though data in children remain mixed (Powe et al., 2013).

Moreover, insulin resistance and hyperinsulinemia, frequently present in pediatric obesity, may influence DBP expression and degradation, further complicating assessment of vitamin D status (Holick et al., 2011).

These changes raise important questions about the adequacy of relying solely on total serum 25(OH)D levels to diagnose deficiency in overweight children. A more nuanced approach, incorporating measures of free or bioavailable vitamin D, may improve diagnostic accuracy in this population.

By revealing the nuance of transport and free fractions, these studies remind us that adequacy is not merely about totals in

the blood, but about the accessibility of those molecules to the tissues that need them.
Such complexities make clear that "true deficiency" is not adequately captured by conventional assays, and that future diagnostics must evolve in line with advances in pediatric endocrinology.

Clinical Implications: Bone Health and Beyond

Vitamin D deficiency in children with obesity carries implications beyond bone health. While low vitamin D is associated with impaired calcium absorption and increased risk of rickets, its consequences extend to musculoskeletal fitness, immune function, and cardiometabolic outcomes.

Musculoskeletal studies show that obese children often have greater bone mass due to mechanical loading, but paradoxically higher risk of fractures, possibly mediated by poor vitamin D status and altered bone quality (Leonard et al., 2015; Foo et al., 2009).

Moreover, several pediatric studies have linked low vitamin D concentrations in obese children with increased risk of insulin resistance, hypertension, and dyslipidemia (Belenchia et al., 2013; Kelly et al., 2011). While causality remains under debate, these associations highlight the systemic consequences of hidden vitamin D deficiency in the context of obesity.

For overweight children, then, low vitamin D is not an isolated lab result but a thread woven into a broader tapestry of skeletal fragility and metabolic vulnerability.
In clinical practice, this means deficiency should be read not as a nutrient anomaly, but as a signal of broader endocrine imbalance with multi-systemic consequences.

Diagnostic Challenges

A major challenge in clinical practice lies in accurately diagnosing vitamin D deficiency in overweight children. Current guidelines use fixed thresholds for serum 25(OH)D (e.g., <50 nmol/L as insufficient), without accounting for differences in body composition or metabolism (Holick et al., 2011). This "one-size-fits-all" approach risks underestimating deficiency in obese children, who may require higher circulating concentrations to achieve functional sufficiency at the tissue level.

Furthermore, conventional assays measure total 25(OH)D but do not account for alterations in DBP or free vitamin D fractions. As Devulapalli (2025) highlight, a paradigm shift toward mechanism-based diagnostics may be necessary to bridge the gap between biochemical adequacy and physiological sufficiency.

Incorporating free or bioavailable vitamin D assays into clinical practice may improve detection of true deficiency in overweight children, guiding more precise treatment.

Recognizing these blind spots may be the first step toward a paradigm where assessments are tailored not to the average child, but to the body before us in the clinic.
This evolving diagnostic landscape highlights how precision medicine principles are increasingly necessary in addressing vitamin D deficiency within obesity.

Supplementation Strategies: Toward Individualized Dosing

Given the altered metabolism and bioavailability of vitamin D in overweight children, conventional supplementation protocols may be inadequate. Several interventional studies suggest that obese children require higher doses of vitamin D to achieve target serum 25(OH)D concentrations compared with their lean peers (Mansbach et al., 2009; Belenchia et al., 2013).

For instance, studies in school-aged children found that standard supplementation regimens (400–600 IU/day) often failed to normalize serum 25(OH)D levels in those with obesity, while higher doses (2,000 IU/day or more) were more effective without evidence of toxicity (Corsello et al., 2023). These findings underscore the need for individualized dosing protocols, guided by body weight, BMI, and potentially inflammatory or metabolic markers.

Personalized dosing regimens informed by patient-specific factors such as BMI, metabolic status, and inflammatory markers are likely to optimize outcomes.

What emerges is the clear message that one-size-fits-all dosing is insufficient, and that thoughtful, individualized regimens stand the best chance of restoring balance. From a policy perspective, this means clinical guidelines should evolve to include weight-adjusted dosing recommendations, ensuring equity in outcomes between normal-weight and overweight children.

Future Directions and Research Gaps

Despite advances, significant gaps remain. Few randomized controlled trials have been conducted specifically in obese children, and optimal dosing strategies are not well established. There is also limited understanding of how vitamin D interacts with obesity-related comorbidities, such as insulin resistance and fatty liver disease, in pediatric populations.

Research into novel biomarkers—such as free vitamin D or tissue-level receptor activity—may provide more precise tools for diagnosis and treatment monitoring.
Longitudinal studies will be critical to determine not only short-term biochemical improvements but also whether correcting vitamin D deficiency alters trajectories of obesity-related diseases into adulthood.

Conclusion

The story of vitamin D in overweight children is, ultimately, one of complexity written into biology itself: fat, inflammation, metabolism, and genetics all conspire to make sufficiency harder to reach.

Vitamin D deficiency in overweight and obese children represents more than inadequate diet or sunlight exposure. It reflects a multifactorial process involving adipose tissue sequestration, altered hepatic metabolism, chronic inflammation, and potential disruptions in vitamin D–binding and receptor signaling.

As highlighted by Devulapalli (2025) and others, this functional deficiency challenges traditional diagnostic and therapeutic approaches. Clinicians should be cautious when interpreting serum 25(OH)D concentrations in children with obesity and should consider higher supplementation doses tailored to body size and metabolic status.

More research, particularly randomized trials in pediatric populations, is urgently needed to define optimal diagnostic markers and supplementation strategies. Until then, a personalized, mechanism-based approach offers the most promising path to improving vitamin D status and overall health in this vulnerable group.
Ultimately, addressing vitamin D deficiency in childhood obesity requires a dual approach: individualized care at the

bedside and forward-looking research that reshapes the diagnostic and therapeutic landscape for future generations.

References

1. Belenchia AM, et al. Correcting vitamin D insufficiency improves insulin sensitivity in obese adolescents: a randomized controlled trial. Am J Clin Nutr. 2013.

2. Blum M, et al. Vitamin D(3) in fat tissue. Endocrine. 2008.

3. Carrelli A, et al. Vitamin D storage in adipose tissue of obese and normal weight women. J Bone Miner Res. 2017.

4. Corsello A, et al. Effects of vitamin D supplementation in obese and overweight children and adolescents: A systematic review and meta-analysis. Pharmacol Res. 2023.

5. Devulapalli CS. Uncovering hidden vitamin D deficiency in overweight children. World J Clin Pediatr 2025; 14(4): 110357.

6. Fiamenghi VI, et al. Vitamin D deficiency in children and adolescents with obesity: a meta-analysis. J Pediatr (Rio J). 2021.

7. Foo LH, et al. Low vitamin D status has an adverse influence on bone mass, bone turnover, and muscle strength in Chinese adolescent girls. J Nutr. 2009.

8. Holick MF, et al. Evaluation, treatment, and prevention of vitamin D deficiency: Endocrine Society guideline. J Clin Endocrinol Metab. 2011.

9. Kelly A, et al. A cross-sectional study of vitamin D and insulin resistance in children. Arch Dis Child. 2011.

10. Leonard MB, et al. Obesity during childhood and adolescence augments bone mass and bone dimensions. J Clin Endocrinol Metab. 2015.

11. Mansbach JM, et al. Serum 25-hydroxyvitamin D levels among US children aged 1 to 11 years: do children need more vitamin D? Pediatrics. 2009.

12. Powe CE, et al. Vitamin D–binding protein and vitamin D status of black Americans and white Americans. N Engl J Med. 2013.

13. Rajakumar K, et al. Vitamin D status, adiposity, and lipids in black American and Caucasian children. J Clin Endocrinol Metab. 2011.

14. Roth CL, et al. Vitamin D deficiency in obese children and its relationship to insulin resistance and adipokines. J Obes. 2011.

15. Turer CB, et al. Prevalence of vitamin D deficiency among overweight and obese US children. Pediatrics. 2013.

16. Vimaleswaran KS, et al. Causal relationship between obesity and vitamin D status: Bi-directional Mendelian randomization analysis. PLoS Med. 2013.

17. Wortsman J, et al. Decreased bioavailability of vitamin D in obesity. Am J Clin Nutr. 2000.

Part III – Vitamin D in Pediatric Immune Function and Disease

8. Immune Pathways to Vitamin D Deficiency in Children

Introduction

Vitamin D deficiency in children has traditionally been explained by insufficient sunlight exposure, inadequate dietary intake, or malabsorption syndromes. These factors undoubtedly play a role, but they do not fully explain the disproportionately high rates of deficiency observed in children with chronic inflammatory and autoimmune conditions. Devulapalli (2025) highlights the importance of moving beyond nutrition and sunlight to consider immune-mediated mechanisms that impair vitamin D metabolism. This new perspective not only reshapes our understanding of vitamin D deficiency in pediatrics but also has direct implications for diagnosis, monitoring, and treatment.

This shift in focus—from passive deficiency to active immune interference—transforms vitamin D from a static nutrient into a dynamic participant in the immunological landscape of childhood.

In this reframing, deficiency is less an issue of scarcity and more a reflection of pathogenic processes that actively distort vitamin D biology, making sufficiency harder to achieve even under otherwise adequate exposures.

Epidemiological Observations in Children

Studies across diverse populations demonstrate that vitamin D deficiency is particularly pronounced in children with autoimmune diseases and chronic inflammatory disorders. For example, children with type 1 diabetes often present with lower serum 25-hydroxyvitamin D [25(OH)D] concentrations than their peers, even after accounting for sunlight exposure and dietary intake (Bener et al., 2012; Zabeen et al., 2022). Similar findings have been reported in juvenile idiopathic arthritis (JIA), where vitamin D insufficiency appears to be common and persistent, irrespective of nutrition or season (Pelajo et al., 2012; Stagi et al., 2014).

Children with inflammatory bowel disease (IBD) also exhibit disproportionately high rates of vitamin D deficiency, even in regions with abundant sunlight exposure. This has been linked not only to malabsorption but also to inflammation-driven alterations in vitamin D metabolism (Pappa et al., 2006; Kim et al., 2019). Likewise, pediatric systemic lupus erythematosus (SLE) is consistently associated with profound vitamin D insufficiency, raising questions about whether immune-mediated mechanisms are central to the deficiency observed in these patients (Lupu et al., 2024).

These patterns suggest that immune-mediated dysregulation contributes to vitamin D deficiency, creating a feedback loop in which inflammation both results from and perpetuates altered vitamin D metabolism.

Across these conditions, the common thread is unmistakable: inflammation reshapes the vitamin D axis in ways that defy sunlight and diet alone.
In other words, deficiency in these contexts is not incidental but integral—woven into the disease process itself.

Mechanisms of Immune-Mediated Vitamin D Deficiency

The pathways by which immune activity interferes with vitamin D homeostasis are increasingly well characterized, though many questions remain.

One central mechanism involves inflammatory cytokines. Chronic immune activation drives elevated production of cytokines such as tumor necrosis factor-α (TNF-α), interleukin-6 (IL-6), and interleukin-1β, which directly alter vitamin D metabolism. Adams & Hewison (2010) demonstrated that these cytokines upregulate the enzyme CYP24A1, responsible for degrading active 1,25-dihydroxyvitamin D, and at the same time suppress CYP27B1, which converts 25(OH)D to its active form. This dual effect leads to accelerated inactivation and impaired activation, leaving the child in a state of relative functional deficiency even if substrate levels appear adequate.

Immune Activation and Vitamin D Status

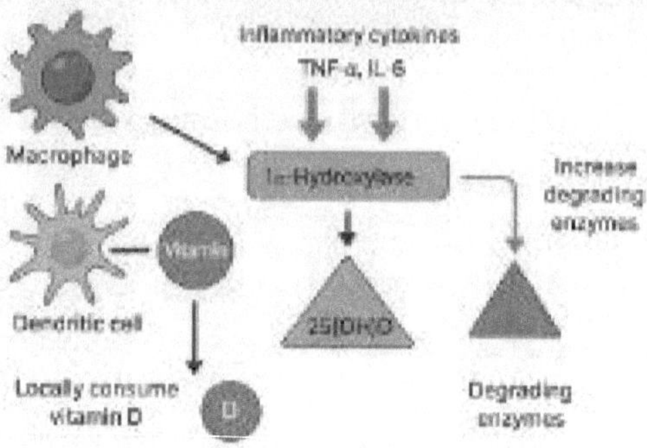

Sîrbe et al. (2022) and Rosli et al. (2025) have further emphasized that immune-mediated pathways may reduce vitamin D receptor (VDR) expression or alter vitamin D–binding protein dynamics, blunting the immunomodulatory effects of vitamin D at the cellular level.

Immune Activation and Vitamin D Metabolism

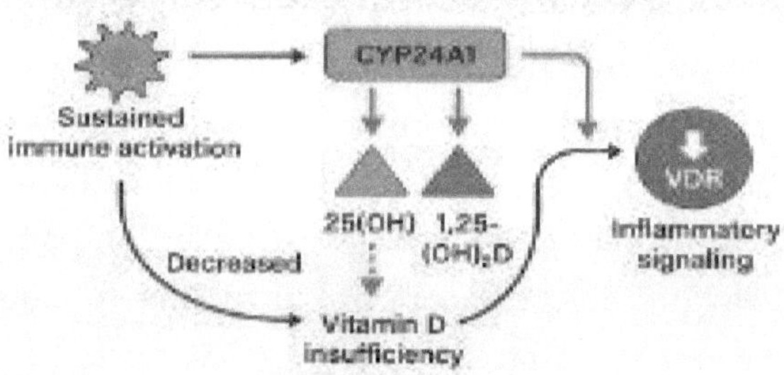

Vitamin D insufficiency

Autoimmune diseases also contribute by altering tissue-level vitamin D handling. In children with type 1 diabetes, inflamed pancreatic islets may overexpress CYP24A1, leading to local degradation of active vitamin D metabolites and reduced paracrine signaling (Zabeen et al., 2022). In juvenile arthritis, inflamed synovial tissue may similarly sequester vitamin D metabolites in a way that limits systemic bioavailability (Stagi et al., 2014). Pediatric IBD presents another mechanistic example: inflamed intestinal tissue exhibits altered expression of both CYP27B1 and CYP24A1, suggesting that inflammation not only impairs absorption but also reshapes vitamin D metabolism within the gut mucosa (Pappa et al., 2006; Kim et al., 2019). In pediatric SLE, immune complexes and persistent cytokine activation appear to reduce both circulating and bioavailable vitamin D (Lupu et al., 2024).

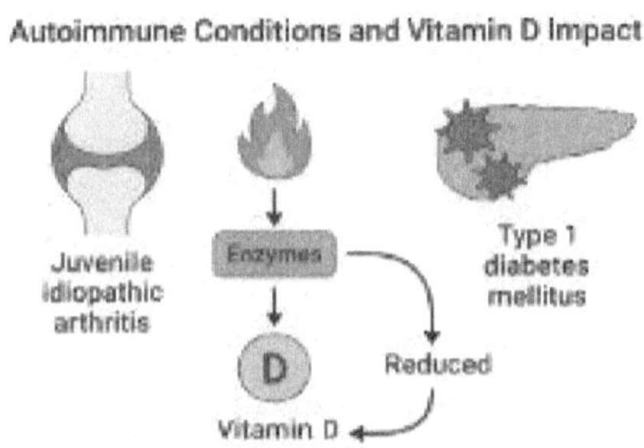

Genetic and epigenetic factors add an additional layer of complexity. Variants in genes encoding the vitamin D receptor (VDR), vitamin D–binding protein (GC), and the key metabolic enzymes CYP27B1 and CYP24A1 have been linked to both lower circulating vitamin D levels and increased susceptibility to autoimmune disease. Hyppönen et al. (2001) provided early evidence of this link in type 1 diabetes, while newer reviews highlight epigenetic regulation in endocrine and autoimmune disorders (Rosli et al., 2025).

As Devulapalli (2025) underscores, the interplay between immune activation and vitamin D metabolism requires a shift in how clinicians think about deficiency. The focus must expand from lifestyle assessment alone to integrated evaluation that considers inflammatory status, genetic background, and disease-specific pathways.
This immunological modulation results in a dynamic deficiency that may not fully respond to standard supplementation, underscoring the need for integrated immune and endocrine management.

In effect, the immune system does not merely suffer the consequences of low vitamin D but actively reconfigures its metabolism, making deficiency partly self-perpetuating.
This reframing compels a new clinical logic: vitamin D status should not only be measured but also interpreted in light of immune activation as both a marker and a mediator of ongoing disease.

Clinical Implications

Recognizing immune-mediated vitamin D deficiency has profound clinical implications. Children with autoimmune or chronic inflammatory conditions should be regarded as high-risk groups, even when their lifestyle factors suggest otherwise. Monitoring vitamin D levels in type 1 diabetes,

JIA, pediatric IBD, and SLE is increasingly seen as part of comprehensive care. Supplementation, while often necessary, may not be sufficient in all cases. Some children may require higher doses, closer monitoring, or adjunctive anti-inflammatory therapies to optimize vitamin D status and function.

At the same time, the safety profile of vitamin D makes supplementation a low-risk intervention, even when mechanistic uncertainties remain. Clinical experience suggests that correcting deficiency may reduce systemic inflammation, improve bone health, and potentially modulate disease activity, although randomized trials in pediatric populations remain limited.

Regular monitoring and personalized treatment strategies are critical for optimizing vitamin D status and potentially modulating disease activity in these high-risk pediatric populations.

Caring for these children therefore requires more than prescribing tablets or drops; it demands recognition that vitamin D sufficiency is entangled with the broader management of inflammation itself.
Here vitamin D ceases to be a passive supplement and becomes a therapeutic ally—one whose efficacy depends on alignment with immunomodulatory care.

Knowledge Gaps and Research Priorities

Several key gaps remain. More longitudinal studies are needed to determine whether immune-mediated vitamin D deficiency precedes autoimmune disease onset or arises as a consequence of disease. Intervention trials should test whether correcting deficiency modifies the course of autoimmune conditions in children, particularly in high-prevalence settings. Advances in genetic and epigenetic profiling may also enable precision medicine approaches, tailoring supplementation to those most likely to benefit. Importantly, mechanistic studies at the interface of immunology and endocrinology are essential to disentangle how cytokines, receptors, and enzymes interact in the pediatric context.

Future research should prioritize longitudinal and interventional studies that clarify causality and inform precision medicine approaches integrating immunology and vitamin D biology.

Closing these gaps will mean uniting immunology, endocrinology, and pediatrics—disciplines too often siloed—into shared strategies for prevention and care.

Bringing these worlds together is not merely an academic exercise; it is the path toward interventions that respect both the molecular detail of disease and the lived experience of children.

Conclusion

When viewed through the prism of immunity, vitamin D deficiency in children is no longer a simple shortfall but a dialogue between genes, inflammation, and environment.

Vitamin D deficiency in children cannot be understood solely in terms of inadequate nutrition or sunlight exposure. Chronic inflammation, autoimmune disease, and underlying genetic factors substantially contribute to impaired vitamin D metabolism, creating an immune-mediated form of deficiency that is increasingly recognized in pediatrics. A growing body of evidence from children with type 1 diabetes, JIA, IBD, and SLE supports this paradigm, and the clinical implications are clear: children with chronic immune activation require special attention to vitamin D status.

Moving forward, clinicians and researchers must adopt a more integrated view of vitamin D in child health, one that accounts for the complex interactions between immunity and metabolism. By bridging these domains, it may be possible not only to prevent deficiency but also to mitigate its impact on disease severity and outcomes in children.

In sum, vitamin D deficiency in immune-mediated disease becomes a prism through which to see the inseparability of nutrition, immunity, and chronic childhood health—a lesson with both clinical urgency and global relevance.

References

1. Adams JS, Hewison M. Update in vitamin D. J Clin Endocrinol Metab. 2010.

2. Bener A, et al. Vitamin D deficiency as a strong predictor of asthma in children. Int Arch Allergy Immunol. 2012.

3. Devulapalli CS. Immune-mediated vitamin D deficiency in children: beyond nutrition and sunlight. World J Pediatr. 2025.

4. Hyppönen E, et al. Intake of vitamin D and risk of type 1 diabetes: a birth-cohort study. Lancet. 2001.

5. Kim S, et al. Association of Vitamin D with Inflammatory Bowel Disease Activity in Pediatric Patients. J Korean Med Sci. 2019.

6. Lupu VV, et al. The role of vitamin D in pediatric systemic lupus erythematosus - a double pawn in the immune and microbial balance. Front Immunol. 2024.

7. Mailhot G, et al. Vitamin D and Immunity in Infants and Children. Nutrients. 2020.

8. Pappa HM, et al. Vitamin D status in children and young adults with inflammatory bowel disease. Pediatrics. 2006.

9. Pelajo CF, et al. 25-hydroxyvitamin D levels and juvenile idiopathic arthritis: is there an association with disease activity? Rheumatol Int. 2012.

10. Rosli NFH, et al. A review of vitamin D deficiency and vitamin D receptor polymorphisms in endocrine-related disorders. Clin Exp Pediatr. 2025.

11. Sîrbe C, et al. An Update on the Effects of Vitamin D on the Immune System and Autoimmune Diseases. Int J Mol Sci. 2022.

12. Stagi S, et al. Determinants of vitamin D levels in children, adolescents, and young adults with juvenile idiopathic arthritis. J Rheumatol. 2014.

13. Zabeen B, et al. Vitamin D status in children and adolescents with type 1 diabetes in a specialized diabetes care centre in Bangladesh. Endocrinol Diabetes Metab. 2022.

9. Vitamin D in Pediatric Asthma: Evidence and Therapeutic Perspectives

Introduction

Asthma remains a leading chronic respiratory condition among children worldwide, characterized by airway inflammation, bronchoconstriction, and variable airflow obstruction. The increasing prevalence of pediatric asthma has prompted extensive research into modifiable risk factors, with vitamin D emerging as a potential contributor. Vitamin D's role extends beyond bone health; it is integral to immune system regulation, influencing both innate and adaptive immune responses. Recent Editorial by Devulapalli (2025) provides a comprehensive synthesis of current data linking vitamin D to pediatric asthma, highlighting observational and interventional studies.

Framing vitamin D within the asthma narrative not only broadens our view of airway disease but also positions this micronutrient at the crossroads of immunity, environment, and child health.

This positioning highlights vitamin D not as an adjunct nutrient, but as a potential determinant shaping inflammatory trajectories, clinical outcomes, and therapeutic opportunities in pediatric asthma.

Epidemiological Evidence in Children

Numerous observational studies have documented an association between low serum 25-hydroxyvitamin D [25(OH)D] levels and increased risk of asthma in children (Jat 2017; Han 2017; Litonjua 2020). Seasonal variation in vitamin D, reflecting sunlight exposure, also correlates with asthma exacerbations, suggesting a potential mechanistic link mediated by immune modulation. These associations are consistent across diverse geographic populations and ethnic groups, reinforcing the global relevance of maintaining sufficient vitamin D status.

For instance, a systematic review found that asthmatic children had significantly lower mean 25(OH)D levels compared to non-asthmatic controls (mean difference −9.41 ng/mL, 95% CI −16.57, −2.25) (Jat 2017). Similarly, vitamin D insufficiency was identified as a risk factor for current asthma and wheeze (Han 2017). Geographic and demographic variations further underscore this concern. Higher deficiency rates have been reported among asthmatic children in Korea (Sung 2023) and in India (Anand 2021).

These consistent associations support the hypothesis that maintaining adequate vitamin D status may be a key element in reducing asthma burden globally.

Taken together, these patterns across populations reinforce the idea that vitamin D sufficiency may represent a silent but powerful determinant of respiratory resilience.

Epidemiologically, therefore, vitamin D status functions less as an incidental correlate and more as a potential risk stratifier in pediatric asthma care.

Mechanisms Linking Vitamin D to Asthma Pathophysiology

Vitamin D influences asthma pathophysiology through several mechanisms. It enhances the production of antimicrobial peptides like cathelicidin and defensins, which have direct antimicrobial properties against respiratory pathogens. Additionally, vitamin D modulates immune responses by influencing the differentiation and function of immune cells, promoting a balanced immune response effective against infections. Furthermore, vitamin D may reduce excessive inflammation by modulating cytokine production, thereby preventing tissue damage during infections.

These mechanisms suggest that adequate vitamin D levels could reduce the incidence and severity of viral respiratory tract infections in children, which are common triggers for asthma exacerbations (Wang M 2019; Fedora 2024). Observational studies indicate that children with lower 25(OH)D levels exhibit greater airway inflammation and higher frequency of exacerbations (Hao 2022; Litonjua 2020). Mechanistic insights align with epidemiological findings, supporting a potential causal relationship.

Thus, vitamin D emerges not merely as a supporting element, but as a potential immunological moderator—quietly narrowing the gap between infection and exacerbation. This dual role—antimicrobial and anti-inflammatory—places vitamin D at a strategic node in asthma pathophysiology, mediating both triggers and downstream inflammatory cascades.

Interventional Evidence and Randomized Trials

Randomized controlled trials examining vitamin D supplementation in pediatric asthma have shown mixed but increasingly positive results. Supplementation appears to reduce the risk of severe exacerbations and improve asthma control in children with insufficient baseline vitamin D (Forno 2020; Wang Q 2022). Benefits are greatest when supplementation targets children with baseline deficiency.

For example, the Vitamin D to Prevent Severe Asthma Exacerbations (VDKA) trial reported that vitamin D supplementation did not significantly alter time to severe exacerbation in children with low vitamin D (Forno 2020), whereas a meta-analysis concluded that supplementation increased serum levels but did not improve asthma control (Hao 2022). In contrast, other systematic reviews and trials observed improvements in exacerbation frequency and FEV1 (Fedora 2024; Wang M 2019).

Discrepancies may stem from differences in study design, participant characteristics, baseline vitamin D levels, dosing, and outcome measures. These variations emphasize the critical need for standardized protocols and well-powered studies to clarify supplementation efficacy across diverse pediatric populations.

These discrepancies remind us that science rarely yields uniform answers, yet the persistence of benefit signals across varied trials argues for continued exploration rather than dismissal.
The heterogeneity of trial results underscores the methodological challenge: supplementation is most effective when deficiency is clearly defined, dosing is optimized, and endpoints are clinically relevant.

Clinical Implications

Given the association between vitamin D deficiency and asthma severity, assessing vitamin D status is advisable in children with recurrent or severe asthma, particularly for those with limited sun exposure, darker skin pigmentation, obesity, or restricted dietary intake. Supplementation should be individualized, aiming for serum 25(OH)D concentrations within recommended ranges, with monitoring for safety (Devulapalli 2025; Kumar 2022).

Optimal dosing remains uncertain, but studies suggest higher doses may more effectively raise serum 25(OH)D. For instance, the VDKA trial administered 4000 IU/day of vitamin D3. However, the clinical significance of increased levels in the absence of clear improvements in outcomes requires cautious interpretation. Potential adverse effects, including hypercalcemia, should be monitored.

Clinicians should balance potential benefits with careful monitoring, especially when considering high-dose supplementation in children with severe or recurrent asthma.

In practice, the conversation about vitamin D and asthma is less about universal prescriptions and more about context—who benefits most, and under which circumstances.
Thus, the clinical lesson is pragmatic: vitamin D should be integrated into asthma care not indiscriminately, but conditionally—based on baseline status, phenotype, and comorbid vulnerability.

Knowledge Gaps and Research Priorities

Despite the growing body of evidence, several critical questions remain regarding the role of vitamin D in pediatric asthma. The optimal dosing strategy for vitamin D supplementation in asthmatic children requires further investigation, including determining the most effective dosage and duration of treatment (Jat 2017; Wang Q 2022). Additionally, the long-term effects of vitamin D supplementation on asthma outcomes, including lung function and exacerbation frequency, are not well understood.

Potential interactions between vitamin D supplementation and other asthma therapies, such as inhaled corticosteroids, need to be explored to understand any synergistic or antagonistic effects (Kumar 2022). Studies examining the impact of vitamin D on airway remodeling could provide insights into its potential role in modifying disease progression.

Mechanistic studies are needed to clarify how vitamin D interacts with airway epithelial cells and the microbiome to modulate asthma risk (Litonjua 2020; Fedora 2024). Research should also focus on identifying subgroups of children who may benefit most from vitamin D supplementation, such as those with specific genetic profiles, comorbid conditions, or environmental exposures. Personalized approaches to supplementation could enhance therapeutic outcomes and minimize unnecessary interventions.

Answering these questions could transform vitamin D from an adjunct consideration into a key therapeutic ally, reshaping how we approach chronic airway disease in children.

Future directions should emphasize precision supplementation—matching dose and duration to phenotype and environment, rather than applying broad-brush strategies.

Conclusion

Ultimately, the story of vitamin D in pediatric asthma is one of promise and complexity: abundant associations, plausible mechanisms, yet the need for precision in application.

Vitamin D deficiency is common among children with asthma and may contribute to greater disease severity and more frequent exacerbations. Observational studies consistently suggest an association between low vitamin D status and asthma outcomes, whereas interventional trials have produced mixed findings regarding the benefits of supplementation. Given its favorable safety profile and potential immunomodulatory effects, vitamin D supplementation may be considered for children with asthma who are deficient, particularly those with recognized risk factors.

Clinicians should tailor supplementation to individual patient needs, balancing possible benefits with careful monitoring. Further well-designed trials are required to determine optimal dosing strategies, clarify long-term outcomes, and identify subgroups most likely to benefit. Until stronger evidence emerges, a personalized and evidence-informed approach remains the most appropriate clinical strategy.

In essence, vitamin D in pediatric asthma represents a frontier of translational medicine—where nutrition, immunology, and respiratory health converge, offering both opportunity and caution in equal measure.

References

1. Anand V, et al. Childhood asthma and vitamin D: case-control study in an academic tertiary care hospital. J Pediatr Res. 2021.

2. Brustad N, et al. Vitamin D primary prevention of respiratory infections and asthma. J Allergy Clin Immunol Pract. 2024.

3. Devulapalli CS. Vitamin D and asthma in pediatrics: evidence and clinical implications. World J Pediatr. 2025.

4. Fedora K, et al. Vitamin D supplementation decrease asthma exacerbations in children: a systematic review and meta-analysis of randomized controlled trials. Ann Med. 2024.

5. Forno E, et al. Effect of vitamin D3 supplementation on severe asthma exacerbations in children with asthma and low vitamin D levels: The VDKA randomized clinical trial. JAMA. 2020.

6. Han YY, et al. Vitamin D Insufficiency and Asthma in a US Nationwide Study. J Allergy Clin Immunol Pract. 2017.

7. Hao M, et al. The effect of vitamin D supplementation in children with asthma: a systematic review and meta-analysis. Front Pediatr. 2022.

8. Jat KR, et al. Vitamin D and asthma in children: A systematic review and meta-analysis of observational studies. Lung India. 2017.

9. Kumar J, et al. Vitamin D supplementation in childhood asthma: a systematic review and meta-analysis of randomised controlled trials. ERJ Open Res. 2021

10. Li W, et al. The correlation between neonatal vitamin D levels and the risk of childhood asthma attacks. Transl Pediatr. 2021.

11. Litonjua AA, et al. Six-Year Follow-up of a Trial of Antenatal Vitamin D for Asthma Reduction. N Engl J Med. 2020.

12. Sharif A, et al. Association of 25-hydroxy vitamin D with asthma and its severity. Clin Mol Allergy. 2020.

13. Sung M, et al. Trends of vitamin D in asthma in the pediatric population for two decades: a systematic review. Clin Exp Pediatr. 2023.

14. Wang M, et al. Association between vitamin D status and asthma control: A meta-analysis of randomized trials. Respir Med. 2019.

15. Wang Q, et al. Vitamin D and asthma occurrence in children: A systematic review and meta-analysis. J Pediatr Nurs. 2022.

10. Immunomodulatory Effects of Vitamin D on Viral Respiratory Infections in Children

Introduction

Viral respiratory tract infections (RTIs) are a leading cause of morbidity in children worldwide. Emerging evidence suggests that vitamin D, through its immunomodulatory effects, may play a significant role in reducing the incidence and severity of these infections. This chapter examines the current literature on the relationship between vitamin D status and viral RTIs in pediatric populations, with a focus on randomized controlled trials (RCTs) and systematic reviews (Devulapalli, 2025; Marusca et al., 2023).

This reframing positions vitamin D not only as a skeletal nutrient but also as a subtle guardian of respiratory resilience in childhood.
This broader perspective reflects a paradigm shift in pediatrics, where micronutrients are increasingly valued as regulators of immune ecosystems, not merely as correctors of dietary deficiencies.

Vitamin D and Immune System Modulation

Vitamin D exerts its effects on the immune system by binding to the vitamin D receptor (VDR), which is expressed on various immune cells, including monocytes, macrophages, dendritic cells, and T lymphocytes. Activation of VDR influences the production of antimicrobial peptides, such as cathelicidin and defensins, which play a crucial role in the innate immune defense against pathogens (Xiao et al., 2021). Additionally, vitamin D modulates the Th1/Th2 balance, promoting a Th1-dominant response that is beneficial in combating viral infections. These immunomodulatory mechanisms provide a foundation for targeted supplementation strategies aimed at enhancing both innate and adaptive immunity in children at risk of RTIs.

In this way, vitamin D provides the immune system with both sharper defenses and gentler regulation, strengthening children's ability to resist infection without inviting excessive inflammation.
This capacity to simultaneously enhance defense and temper inflammatory harm explains why vitamin D is uniquely suited to modulate viral infection outcomes in developing immune systems.

Mechanisms of Action

The protective effects of vitamin D against viral respiratory tract infections are mediated through multiple, interconnected mechanisms. Vitamin D enhances innate immunity by upregulating the production of antimicrobial peptides, such as cathelicidin and defensins, which exert direct antimicrobial activity against a broad spectrum of respiratory pathogens (Walker et al., 2009). At the same time, it modulates adaptive immune responses by influencing the differentiation and function of various immune cells, thereby promoting a balanced response that is both effective in combating infections and protective against immune overactivation. Furthermore, vitamin D contributes to the regulation of inflammatory pathways, tempering cytokine production to reduce excessive inflammation that can otherwise cause tissue damage during infection. Together, these mechanisms underscore the multifaceted role of vitamin D in shaping immune function and its potential in preventing and mitigating viral respiratory infections in children.

These converging pathways reveal vitamin D as less a single trigger than a conductor, orchestrating balance between innate defense, adaptive precision, and inflammatory restraint.
By operating across multiple checkpoints of immunity, vitamin D emerges less as a supplement and more as a biological moderator capable of stabilizing fragile pediatric immune networks.

Epidemiological Evidence in Children

Several studies have documented an association between low serum 25-hydroxyvitamin D [25(OH)D] concentrations and increased susceptibility to viral RTIs in children (Esposito et al., 2015; Devulapalli, 2025). For instance, children with viral upper respiratory tract infections often present with lower vitamin D concentrations, and supplementation frequently reduces the risk of infection (Devulapalli, 2025). Similarly, systematic reviews indicate that vitamin D supplementation may lower RTI incidence in children, particularly those with baseline deficiency (Marusca et al., 2023). Observational associations are supported by growing interventional data, underscoring the need to consider baseline vitamin D status when tailoring supplementation.

What emerges is a consistent picture: deficiency is not just a laboratory finding but a shadow that lengthens the risk of respiratory illness across diverse pediatric populations. These population patterns move the conversation from individual variability toward public health urgency, where deficiency signals elevated vulnerability across whole pediatric cohorts.

Randomized Controlled Trials and Meta-Analyses

Randomized controlled trials (RCTs) have provided robust evidence for vitamin D supplementation in preventing viral RTIs. A meta-analysis of 37 RCTs found that supplementation significantly reduced the incidence of acute respiratory infections in children, with the greatest benefit in those with baseline 25(OH)D concentrations <25 nmol/L (Jolliffe et al., 2021). Importantly, the seminal individual participant data meta-analysis by Martineau et al. (2017) reported a protective effect of vitamin D against acute respiratory tract infections overall, with strongest benefit seen in those with profound deficiency and in trials using daily or weekly dosing without bolus supplementation.

In contrast, Aglipay et al. (2017) reported that high-dose vitamin D did not prevent wintertime viral RTIs in healthy children, emphasizing the importance of baseline deficiency and individualized dosing. Other RCTs highlight similar nuances: Loeb et al. (2019) and Xiao et al. (2021) demonstrated reductions in infection risk and improved immune parameters, particularly in children with recurrent RTIs or low baseline vitamin D.

Recent pediatric trials and analyses further strengthen these findings. Reyes et al. (2024) reported that weekly vitamin D supplementation reduced RTI incidence in young children across multiple latitudes, while Binks et al. (2023) showed benefit in First Nations infants using perinatal vitamin D. Brustad et al. (2024) highlighted the preventive potential of vitamin D in early-life RTIs and asthma. Tanase et al. (2024) and Marusca et al. (2023) similarly report improvements in respiratory outcomes with supplementation in deficient children. Taken together, these studies indicate that vitamin D supplementation is most effective when baseline deficiency is corrected, dosing is adequate, and high-risk pediatric populations are targeted.

Across these varied trials, one truth consistently surfaces: correction of profound deficiency carries the most promise, underscoring the importance of targeting those most at risk.

This recurring theme provides a practical clinical maxim: measure, identify, and treat deficiency early, particularly in children most biologically or socio-environmentally vulnerable.

Clinical Implications

Given this evidence, clinicians should assess vitamin D status in children at risk of deficiency, particularly during winter or in populations with limited sun exposure (Esposito et al., 2015; Walker et al., 2009). Supplementation may be warranted in deficient children to reduce RTI incidence and severity (Devulapalli, 2025; Marusca et al., 2023).

Public health strategies could include fortification of foods with vitamin D and recommendations for safe sunlight exposure. Healthcare providers should consider potential interactions between vitamin D and medications such as corticosteroids that may influence vitamin D metabolism (Xiao et al., 2021). Incorporating vitamin D assessment into routine pediatric care for vulnerable groups can inform evidence-based supplementation decisions and reduce RTI-related morbidity globally.

Thus, evaluation of vitamin D status offers clinicians a tangible lever—simple to measure, safe to correct—with potential impact on the everyday burden of pediatric infections.

Incorporating this practice not only addresses individual health but also aligns with broader systems-level goals of reducing healthcare use, hospitalizations, and school absences driven by preventable infections.

Knowledge Gaps and Research Priorities

Despite compelling evidence supporting vitamin D's immunomodulatory role, several critical gaps remain. First, the optimal dosing strategies, timing, and duration of supplementation across different pediatric age groups and risk profiles are not fully established (Jolliffe et al., 2021; Reyes et al., 2024), limiting precise clinical recommendations. Second, there is limited longitudinal data assessing the long-term effects of vitamin D sufficiency on immune development and resilience against recurrent infections (Esposito et al., 2015). Third, most studies have focused on otherwise healthy children; evidence is sparse regarding high-risk populations, including children with chronic illnesses, obesity, or immunodeficiency, in whom the immunomodulatory effects of vitamin D may differ (Walker et al., 2009; Xiao et al., 2021). Finally, mechanistic insights linking specific 25(OH)D thresholds to cellular and molecular antiviral responses in pediatric populations are incomplete (Jolliffe et al., 2021; Devulapalli, 2025), constraining our understanding of causality.

Future research should address these gaps by conducting well-designed randomized trials, mechanistic studies, and population-based analyses across diverse pediatric cohorts, exploring both clinical effectiveness and immune endpoints (Marusca et al., 2023; Tanase et al., 2024). Such work will be critical to refine guidelines and translate current knowledge into effective, evidence-based prevention strategies.

Closing these gaps will allow us to move beyond hopeful correlations toward precise interventions, where dose, timing, and target population align for maximum protection. Bridging these research divides will require collaboration between pediatrics, immunology, and public health policy, transforming vitamin D into not just a nutrient of interest but a cornerstone of preventive child health.

Conclusion

Ultimately, the story of vitamin D and viral infections in childhood illustrates how a micronutrient can act as both shield and signal, quietly shaping respiratory health on a global scale.

Vitamin D plays a significant role in modulating the immune system and enhancing the body's defense against viral respiratory tract infections in children (Walker et al., 2009; Devulapalli, 2025). While supplementation appears beneficial, particularly in those with low baseline levels, further research is needed to determine optimal dosing strategies and to understand the long-term effects of vitamin D supplementation on immune function and overall health in the pediatric population (Jolliffe et al., 2021; Marusca et al., 2023).

Vitamin D assessment and supplementation represent actionable strategies to reduce the burden of viral respiratory tract infections in children worldwide. Clinicians can integrate routine evaluation of serum 25(OH)D levels into pediatric care, particularly for high-risk populations such as children with limited sun exposure, darker skin pigmentation, or chronic comorbidities (Esposito et al., 2015; Xiao et al., 2021). Evidence-based supplementation protocols, informed by baseline vitamin D status, season, and geographic latitude, have the potential to improve infection outcomes, reduce healthcare utilization, and support overall pediatric health.

For scientists and policy makers, these findings highlight the need for harmonized guidelines on vitamin D sufficiency for immune health, beyond traditional bone outcomes (Tanase et al., 2024; Reyes et al., 2024). Public health initiatives—including dietary fortification, safe sun exposure campaigns, and population-targeted supplementation programs—could mitigate seasonal and geographic disparities in vitamin D status and susceptibility to viral RTIs. Future research should prioritize large, multicenter trials across diverse pediatric cohorts to refine dosing strategies, quantify population-level benefits, and inform global policies that optimize child health outcomes.

In closing, vitamin D's role in reducing viral RTI burden among children underscores a larger lesson in pediatrics: that small, cost-effective interventions targeting common deficiencies can yield substantial global health dividends.

References

1. Aglipay M, et al. Effect of high-dose vs standard-dose wintertime vitamin D supplementation on viral upper

respiratory tract infections in young healthy children. JAMA. 2017.

2. Binks MJ, et al. Randomised controlled trial of perinatal vitamin D supplementation to prevent early-onset acute respiratory infections among Australian First Nations infants. BMJ Open Respir Res. 2023.

3. Brustad N, et al. Vitamin D primary prevention of respiratory infections and asthma: a systematic review. J Allergy Clin Immunol Pract. 2024.

4. Devulapalli CS. Vitamin D supplements reduce risk of viral upper respiratory infections in children with lower concentrations. Acta Paediatr. 2025.

5. Esposito S, et al. Vitamin D and respiratory tract infections in childhood. BMC Infect Dis. 2015.

6. Jeyakumar A, et al. Effect of vitamin D supplementation on the immune response to respiratory infections in children. Human Nutrition and Metabolism. 2024.

7. Jolliffe DA, et al. Vitamin D supplementation to prevent acute respiratory infections: a systematic review and meta-analysis of aggregate data from randomised controlled trials. Lancet Diabetes Endocrinol. 2021.

8. Lee MT, et al. Randomized phase 2 trial of monthly vitamin D to prevent respiratory infections in children. Blood Adv. 2018.

9. Loeb M, et al. Effect of Vitamin D supplementation to reduce respiratory infections in children: a randomized trial. Influenza Other Respir Viruses. 2019.

10. Martineau AR, et al. Vitamin D supplementation to prevent acute respiratory tract infections: systematic review and meta-analysis of individual participant data. BMJ. 2017.

11. Marusca LM, et al. The Effects of Vitamin D Supplementation on Respiratory Infections in Children under 6 Years Old: A Systematic Review. J Pediatr Health. 2023.

12. Reyes ML, et al. Weekly Vitamin D Supplementation to Prevent Acute Respiratory Infections in Young Children at Different Latitudes: A Randomized Controlled Trial. J Pediatr. 2024.

13. Sarau OS, et al. Exploring the Preventive Potential of Vitamin D against Respiratory Infections in Preschool-Age Children. Nutrients. 2024.

14. Tanase E, et al. Assessing the Impact of Vitamin D Supplementation on Respiratory Infections in

Children and Adolescents: A Cross-Sectional Study. Nutrients. 2024.

15. Walker VP, et al. The vitamin D connection to pediatric infections and immune function. Pediatr Res. 2009.

16. Xiao J, et al. The immunomodulatory effects of vitamin D drops in children with recurrent respiratory tract infections. Am J Transl Res. 2021.

11. Vitamin D in Atopic Dermatitis and Allergic Rhinitis

Introduction

Vitamin D, historically recognized for its pivotal role in bone mineralization and calcium-phosphate homeostasis, has emerged over the last two decades as a crucial immunomodulatory hormone. Increasingly, attention has turned to its role in allergic diseases of childhood—particularly atopic dermatitis (AD) and allergic rhinitis (AR)—which represent the earliest manifestations of the atopic march. These conditions, highly prevalent and often coexisting, are driven by complex immune dysregulation and barrier dysfunction, and their rising global burden has intensified interest in modifiable environmental and biological risk factors. Recent evidence, including the review by Devulapalli (2025), suggests that vitamin D may influence both disease onset and severity by modulating skin and mucosal immunity, as well as systemic allergic responses.

By situating vitamin D within the atopic march, we see how a single micronutrient can influence the earliest expressions of allergy, carrying implications that extend well beyond the skin and nose.

In this sense, vitamin D has evolved from a skeletal nutrient to a candidate modifier of the allergic trajectory in children, offering a unifying thread between molecular biology and clinical expression.

Mechanistic Insights: Linking Vitamin D to Allergic Inflammation

Vitamin D acts through the vitamin D receptor (VDR), a nuclear transcription factor expressed in keratinocytes, airway epithelial cells, dendritic cells, T lymphocytes, and B cells (Hewison, 2012). This widespread distribution underscores its broad regulatory potential. In atopic dermatitis, vitamin D contributes to epidermal barrier integrity by enhancing filaggrin expression and ceramide synthesis, thereby reducing transepidermal water loss and allergen penetration (Hata et al., 2008). In parallel, it stimulates antimicrobial peptide production, including cathelicidin (LL-37), providing protection against Staphylococcus aureus, a common colonizer that exacerbates AD flares (Peroni et al., 2011).

In allergic rhinitis, vitamin D modulates dendritic cell maturation, promotes regulatory T cell (Treg) development, and suppresses Th2 cytokine secretion, limiting IgE production and eosinophilic inflammation (Majak et al., 2012; Alyasin et al., 2011). By enhancing mucosal barrier function, vitamin D reduces allergen uptake and subsequent sensitization. Experimental work has also shown that VDR gene polymorphisms influence immune responses and disease expression in both AD and AR, highlighting a potential genetic basis for differential responsiveness (Penna-Martinez et al., 2009).

These molecular effects form the biological basis for the potential clinical benefits observed with vitamin D supplementation in atopic diseases.

Thus, vitamin D touches both the threshold of the body's barriers and the depth of its immune networks, shaping how children experience allergens from their first encounters. This mechanistic reach situates vitamin D as a bridge across immune tolerance, epithelial integrity, and microbial defense—three pillars of allergy regulation.

Epidemiological Evidence in Atopic Dermatitis

Several pediatric observational studies have consistently linked low serum 25-hydroxyvitamin D [25(OH)D] levels to increased risk and severity of AD. Peroni et al., 2011 demonstrated that Italian children with moderate-to-severe AD had significantly lower vitamin D levels compared to controls, particularly in winter months. Similar findings were replicated in Asian populations, suggesting this association is consistent across ethnicities (Samochocki et al., 2013; Lee et al., 2013). Children with AD and concurrent allergic sensitization tend to have the lowest vitamin D levels, supporting the hypothesis that deficiency exacerbates disease in atopy-prone individuals (Miyake et al., 2011). Recent comprehensive reviews further support these associations and emphasize vitamin D's immunomodulatory role in restoring immune balance in AD, particularly via suppression of Th2-mediated inflammation (Zhang et al., 2024; Ng et al, 2025).

Mechanistic RCTs have begun to test supplementation efficacy. Borzutzky et al., 2024 found that weekly vitamin D over six weeks improved serum levels but did not significantly alter SCORAD scores or type 2 immunity biomarkers. Mansour et al., 2020 reported significant clinical improvement in EASI scores when vitamin D was used as an adjuvant to standard therapy. A recent meta-analysis (Ng et al, 2025) confirmed strongest clinical benefits in patients with baseline deficiency and demonstrated dose-dependent efficacy. Meanwhile, meta-analyses highlight heterogeneity with some divergence, reinforcing the need to personalize treatment strategies (Nielsen et al., 2024).

Other interventional studies provide supportive evidence. Javanbakht et al., 2011 demonstrated that supplementation with 2000 IU/day of vitamin D over 12 weeks improved SCORAD indices in children with moderate AD. However, smaller trials in mild disease showed mixed outcomes (Amestejani et al., 2012). Overall, supplementation appears most beneficial in children with baseline deficiency and more severe phenotypes.

The consistency of these findings across diverse populations underscores the global relevance of vitamin D as a modifiable risk factor in AD.

The weight of these converging studies suggests that vitamin D status may serve not just as a marker of disease burden but also as a modifier of clinical trajectory in atopic dermatitis.

Thus, even in a condition classically defined by barrier defects and Th2 skewing, vitamin D surfaces as a pivotal cofactor influencing disease course.

Vitamin D and Allergic Rhinitis

The role of vitamin D in AR has been less extensively studied but is gaining recognition. Cross-sectional surveys have shown inverse associations between serum vitamin D and AR prevalence in children. Camargo et al., 2007 found that maternal vitamin D intake during pregnancy was inversely associated with AR risk in offspring, suggesting possible prenatal programming effects. A Japanese cohort later demonstrated that children with higher serum 25(OH)D had lower prevalence of seasonal AR, particularly pollen-induced rhinitis (Yang et al., 2021). A Turkish pediatric cohort also confirmed that children with both perennial and seasonal AR had lower serum vitamin D compared with healthy peers (Okmen et al., 2021).

Interventional data remain scarce. Majak et al., 2012 conducted an RCT in children with AR and asthma, reporting that vitamin D supplementation enhanced responsiveness to subcutaneous immunotherapy, suggesting an adjuvant role in allergic treatment. Other small pediatric trials have reported symptomatic improvement during pollen season, but variability in dosage and study design limits definitive conclusions (Alyasin et al., 2011). Importantly, these findings align with the mechanistic evidence that vitamin D strengthens mucosal defenses and mitigates Th2-dominated responses in AR.

Emerging evidence for vitamin D's role in AR complements its established immunomodulatory functions, suggesting a broader impact across respiratory allergic diseases.

Together, these findings hint at vitamin D as a quiet mediator of airway balance, tempering seasonal triggers and strengthening defenses where the environment first meets the child's body.
While not yet definitive, this expanding evidence base signals vitamin D as a plausible adjunctive tool in reducing allergic airway morbidity.

Shared Pathophysiology Across Atopic Diseases

A unifying theme across AD and AR is the disruption of epithelial barriers and skewing toward Th2 immune responses. Vitamin D, by modulating barrier function and immune balance, targets both central pathogenic features. Moreover, vitamin D influences the microbiome, which plays a critical role in mucosal and skin homeostasis. Emerging pediatric studies indicate that vitamin D deficiency is associated with reduced microbial diversity, potentially amplifying allergic inflammation (Litonjua & Weiss, 2007; Kamen & Tangpricha, 2010). These insights suggest that adequate vitamin D status may help stabilize epithelial–immune–microbiome interactions, slowing or modifying the trajectory of the allergic march.

Understanding the interactions between vitamin D, barrier integrity, and the microbiome may open new avenues for integrated therapeutic strategies.

Additionally, the global burden of vitamin D deficiency in children with AD and AR underscores its public health significance. Children in higher-latitude regions, those with darker skin pigmentation, or limited outdoor exposure are particularly at risk, suggesting that preventive strategies should be tailored to local environmental and demographic factors. Recognizing these at-risk populations allows clinicians and policymakers to prioritize interventions where they are most likely to reduce disease severity and improve long-term outcomes.

In this light, adequate vitamin D emerges as a common thread capable of weaving resilience into the fragile fabric of epithelial barriers and immune tolerance.
This shared biology invites a broader conceptualization of vitamin D—as a nutritional pivot point influencing the entire trajectory of the allergic march.

Clinical Implications and Challenges

The clinical application of these findings is not straightforward. Vitamin D deficiency is common in children worldwide, particularly in those with limited outdoor exposure or higher skin pigmentation. However, optimal serum levels for allergy prevention or management remain undefined. Current pediatric guidelines focus on bone health, not immune outcomes, and therefore may underestimate requirements for children at risk of allergic disease (Holick et al., 2011).

Preliminary evidence, including the review by Devulapalli (2025), argues for considering phenotype-specific supplementation strategies—particularly in children with moderate-to-severe AD, seasonal AR, or those with coexisting vitamin D deficiency. Still, routine supplementation for allergic disease prevention is not yet supported by definitive trial evidence, and concerns about over-supplementation warrant caution. Stratification by baseline vitamin D status, allergic phenotype, and genetic polymorphisms may be necessary to clarify which children benefit most.

Finally, integrating lifestyle and nutritional measures alongside supplementation may enhance effectiveness. Encouraging safe sun exposure, ensuring dietary intake of vitamin D–rich foods, and monitoring high-risk children can provide a holistic approach. Attention to dosing safety, including adherence to upper limits and biochemical monitoring, ensures interventions are both effective and safe, reinforcing trust in public health recommendations and clinical practice.

Future guideline development should consider stratified supplementation approaches tailored to allergic phenotype, baseline vitamin D status, and genetic predisposition.

What remains, therefore, is not a call for indiscriminate dosing but for strategies that match biology with phenotype, ensuring interventions are as precise as the mechanisms they aim to influence.
Clinicians are thus called to integrate vitamin D management into allergy care with nuance, balancing preventive promise against evidentiary gaps.

Knowledge Gaps and Research Priorities

Key unanswered questions include the optimal timing of intervention (prenatal versus early childhood), appropriate dosage for immune modulation, and long-term safety in higher-risk children. The heterogeneity of trial findings reflects the need for larger, multicenter pediatric RCTs stratified by baseline deficiency and allergic phenotypes. Genetic and epigenetic studies may further elucidate inter-individual variability in response. Another priority is clarifying vitamin D's interaction with the microbiome and allergen immunotherapy, both of which hold promise for integrated treatment approaches.

Answering these questions may allow future clinicians to use vitamin D not only as a supplement, but as a tailored tool for reshaping the allergic march itself.

Bridging these knowledge gaps would elevate vitamin D from supportive care into a precision tool for allergy prevention and modulation.

Conclusion

Seen through the lens of allergy, vitamin D ceases to be merely supportive of bones and becomes a negotiator at the barrier between environment and child.

Vitamin D deficiency is increasingly recognized as a modifiable contributor to pediatric atopic dermatitis and allergic rhinitis. Mechanistic studies highlight its role in epithelial barrier function, antimicrobial defense, and immune modulation, while epidemiological evidence links deficiency to increased prevalence and severity of both conditions. Interventional trials suggest potential symptomatic benefit, particularly in deficient children with severe disease, but results remain inconsistent. Until robust guidelines are established, ensuring adequate vitamin D intake through diet, safe sun exposure, and selective supplementation appears to be a pragmatic strategy for reducing the burden of allergic disease in children.

Ultimately, vitamin D represents a modest intervention with disproportionate potential—capable not only of strengthening bones, but of reshaping the earliest immunological steps in the atopic march.

References

1. Amestejani M et al. Vitamin D supplementation in the treatment of atopic dermatitis: a clinical trial study. J Drugs Dermatol. 2012.

2. Alyasin S et al. Effect of vitamin D supplementation on allergic rhinitis. Iran J Allergy Asthma Immunol. 2011.

3. Borzutzky A et al. Effect of weekly vitamin D supplementation on the severity of atopic dermatitis and type 2 immunity biomarkers in children: A randomized controlled trial. J Eur Acad Dermatol Venereol. 2024.

4. Chakkamadathil JK et al. Vitamin D Levels in Children with Allergic Rhinitis and Asthma in South India: A Cross-Sectional Study. J Adv Lung Health. 2023.

5. Devulapalli CS et al. Modulatory role of vitamin D in atopic dermatitis and allergic rhinitis. World J Clin Pediatr. In press. 2025.

6. Hewison M. Vitamin D and human immunity: update. Clin Endocrinol (Oxf). 2012.

7. Hata TR et al. Administration of oral vitamin D induces cathelicidin production in atopic individuals. J Allergy Clin Immunol. 2008.

8. Holick MF et al. Evaluation, Treatment, and Prevention of Vitamin D Deficiency: an Endocrine

Society Clinical Practice Guideline. J Clin Endocrinol Metab. 2011.

9. Javanbakht MH et al. Randomized controlled trial using vitamins E and D supplementation in atopic dermatitis. J Dermatolog Treat. 2011.

10. Jerzyńska J et al. Clinical and immunological effects of vitamin D supplementation during the pollen season in children with allergic rhinitis. Arch Med Sci. 2018.

11. Kamen DL et al. Vitamin D and immune regulation. J Mol Med. 2010.

12. Majak P et al. Correlation of vitamin D with Foxp3 induction and steroid-sparing effect of immunotherapy in asthmatic children. Ann Allergy Asthma Immunol. 2012.

13. Ng V, et al. The impact of vitamin D on atopic disorders: a meta-analysis. Front Nutr. 2025.

14. Nielsen AY et al. Vitamin D Supplementation for Treating Atopic Dermatitis in Children and Adults: A Systematic Review and Meta-Analysis. Nutrients. 2024.

15. Okmen ZH et al. The Effect of Serum Vitamin D Level on Allergic Rhinitis Symptoms in Children. Pediatr Allergy Immunol Pulmonol. 2021.

16. Penna-Martinez M et al. Vitamin D receptor polymorphisms in differentiated thyroid carcinoma. Thyroid. 2009.

17. Peroni DG et al. Correlation between serum 25-hydroxyvitamin D levels and severity of atopic dermatitis in children. Br J Dermatol. 2011.

18. Samochocki Z et al. Vitamin D effects in atopic dermatitis. J Am Acad Dermatol. 2013.

19. Yang L et al. Serum 25-Hydroxyvitamin D Concentrations and Atopic Dermatitis in Early Childhood: Findings from the Japan Environment and Children's Study. Nutrients. 2021.

20. Zhang P et al. Vitamin D and allergic diseases. Front Immunol. 2024.

12. Fatigue in Childhood: Links to Vitamin D Deficiency

Introduction

Fatigue in children is a common but often under-recognized complaint that impairs quality of life, school attendance, and psychosocial functioning. Pediatric clinicians frequently attribute persistent tiredness to psychosocial stress, sleep disturbance, anemia, or chronic disease; however, mounting evidence suggests that nutritional factors — notably vitamin D insufficiency — may be an underappreciated, reversible contributor in many cases (Devulapalli et al., 2025). Vitamin D deficiency is widespread worldwide, particularly among children with limited sun exposure, darker skin pigmentation, indoor lifestyles, or diets low in fortified foods. Clinicians evaluating children with unexplained fatigue may therefore overlook an opportunity to diagnose and treat hypovitaminosis D, thereby improving symptoms with a simple, low-cost intervention. This chapter synthesizes mechanistic, observational, and interventional evidence to provide a practical framework for assessment and management.

In this reframing, fatigue is not dismissed as vague or psychosomatic, but recognized as a potential signal of nutritional imbalance—one that may be corrected with precision and care.

Placing fatigue in this biomedical context invites clinicians to look beyond psychosocial explanations and to systematically assess reversible metabolic factors such as vitamin D deficiency.

Biological Plausibility: Mechanisms linking Vitamin D to Fatigue

Multiple biological pathways plausibly link low vitamin D status to fatigue. Skeletal muscle expresses vitamin D receptors (VDR) and 1α-hydroxylase, enabling local activation and genomic effects on muscle protein synthesis, calcium handling, and mitochondrial function (Ceglia, 2009). Experimental and translational studies show that correction of vitamin D deficiency improves markers of mitochondrial oxidative phosphorylation and reduces oxidative stress in muscle tissue, mechanisms that plausibly enhance muscular endurance and reduce perceived exertional fatigue (Sinha et al., 2013; Filgueiras et al., 2020). Vitamin D also modulates systemic inflammation: deficiency is associated with higher circulating concentrations of IL-6 and TNF-α, cytokines implicated in central fatigue and sickness behavior (Grudet et al., 2020).

Preclinical and clinical evidence supports interactions with neurotransmitter systems and HPA-axis regulation, which may influence central perception of energy and mood. Together, these pathways support a biologically coherent link between vitamin D and both peripheral (muscle) and central (neuro-immune) components of fatigue.

This multifactorial influence positions vitamin D as a key modifiable factor in both central and peripheral components of pediatric fatigue.

The convergence of muscular, neuro-immune, and inflammatory pathways reveals vitamin D as not merely supportive but integrative—connecting energy, mood, and physical performance in the developing child.
This integrative role underscores the plausibility that fatigue in children may be an early and under-acknowledged marker of hypovitaminosis D.

Epidemiological Evidence in Children

Observational pediatric studies consistently associate lower serum 25-hydroxyvitamin D [25(OH)D] with fatigue-related complaints. Vehapoglu et al. (2015) observed that children with growing pains and low 25(OH)D experienced substantial symptomatic relief after correction of deficiency. Zhang et al. (2020) reported that low vitamin D correlated with lower physical activity and greater reports of tiredness. School-based and community studies in adolescents also link lower 25(OH)D to greater daytime sleepiness and fatigue complaints (Mocayar Marón et al., 2020). Cross-sectional analyses of children with chronic inflammatory conditions show inverse associations between vitamin D status and fatigue measures (Finch et al., 2018; Pappa et al., 2006).

The consistency of these findings across different populations supports vitamin D deficiency as a potential therapeutic target to improve fatigue symptoms.

These consistent associations invite clinicians to view fatigue not just as a nebulous complaint, but as a symptom with a measurable and modifiable biological substrate.

From a public health perspective, these associations argue for routine awareness campaigns targeting vitamin D as a determinant of functional well-being, not just bone health.

Interventional Evidence: Pediatric Trials and Recent Reviews

Randomized controlled trials in children remain limited but provide important insights. Dougherty et al. (2020) found improvements in health-related quality of life and physical performance with 4,000 IU/day supplementation in children with low baseline 25(OH)D. Högberg et al. (2012) reported improved depressive symptoms and reduced fatigue in adolescents receiving 1,500–2,000 IU/day. Vehapoglu et al. (2015) documented meaningful symptom reduction after a high-dose therapeutic regimen in children with growing pains and vitamin D deficiency.

These pediatric trials collectively suggest that vitamin D supplementation can improve fatigue-related outcomes, particularly when deficiency is present. Recent narrative and systematic reviews further emphasize that supplementation has the greatest likelihood of benefit when baseline 25(OH)D is low, dosing is sufficient to achieve adequate serum concentrations, and validated fatigue instruments are used (Di Molfetta et al., 2024; López-Muñoz et al., 2023; Filgueiras et al., 2020).

To strengthen the pediatric evidence base since 2021, several recent publications are noteworthy. Middelkoop et al. (2024), reporting secondary outcomes from the ViDiKids randomized trial, demonstrated that vitamin D supplementation in schoolchildren improved measures of muscle strength and exercise capacity — outcomes mechanistically linked to fatigue. Di Molfetta et al. (2024) provided a comprehensive narrative synthesis across pediatric and adolescent populations, confirming that supplementation tends to reduce fatigue symptoms when deficiency is present, although heterogeneity in design and outcome measurement limits pooled estimates. López-Muñoz et al. (2023) and Filgueiras et al. (2020) reinforce the mechanistic plausibility and clinical relevance of these findings, highlighting improvements in both muscle function and inflammatory markers associated with fatigue.

Taken together, these studies indicate that vitamin D supplementation in children is most effective for improving fatigue when: (a) baseline 25(OH)D is low, (b) dosing is sufficient to raise serum concentrations into the adequate range, and (c) validated, rigorous fatigue instruments are employed.

Nevertheless, variability in trial designs, dosing regimens, and outcome measures necessitates cautious interpretation, highlighting the ongoing need for standardized, high-quality pediatric studies using validated fatigue assessments.

Together, these findings suggest that correcting deficiency can lift the veil of fatigue for many children, transforming a vague symptom into a clear therapeutic target.

The translational message is clear: vitamin D is unlikely to resolve every case of fatigue, but in the context of deficiency, it represents one of the most efficient and low-risk interventions available.

Practical Diagnostic Approach in Children with Unexplained Fatigue

Given the multifactorial nature of pediatric fatigue, vitamin D testing should be targeted rather than universal. Measurement of serum 25(OH)D is appropriate in children presenting with persistent, unexplained fatigue after a basic evaluation, particularly when risk factors are present: darker skin, limited sun exposure, obesity, restrictive diets, or chronic inflammatory disease (Holick et al., 2011; Devulapalli et al., 2025). Most authorities define deficiency as <20 ng/mL (50 nmol/L) and insufficiency as 20–30 ng/mL (50–75 nmol/L). Symptomatic improvement may occur when levels rise above ~30 ng/mL (Holick et al., 2011; Mocayar Marón et al., 2020).

Targeted testing focused on high-risk groups may prevent missed diagnoses and facilitate timely intervention, optimizing quality of life outcomes for affected children.

Such targeted screening respects both biology and clinical pragmatism, ensuring interventions are directed where they matter most.

Integrating fatigue as a potential clinical cue for testing shifts vitamin D from an ancillary check to a core part of pediatric diagnostic reasoning.

Treatment considerations and monitoring

When deficiency is confirmed, cholecalciferol (vitamin D_3) is the preferred preparation. Pediatric trials used daily doses of 1,500–4,000 IU/day or therapeutic bolus regimens tailored to baseline deficiency. Clinicians should individualize dosing by age, weight, baseline concentration, comorbidity, and local guidelines, monitoring serum 25(OH)D and calcium when high or repeated bolus dosing is used (Devulapalli et al., 2025). Correction is generally safe when performed according to recommended protocols, and adverse events are uncommon.

Individualized treatment plans guided by clinical context and biochemical monitoring ensure safe and effective correction of deficiency-related fatigue.

In this way, supplementation becomes not a blanket prescription but a tailored corrective, guided by risk factors, biochemical thresholds, and careful follow-up.
The goal is restoration of functional energy, not merely normalization of laboratory numbers.

Integration with broader evaluation and management

Vitamin D assessment and correction should be part of a holistic approach to fatigue. Sleep hygiene, screening for anemia and thyroid disease, assessment for mood disorders, and evaluation of physical activity and nutrition remain essential (Roy et al., 2014; Głąbska et al., 2021). Addressing vitamin D deficiency may synergize with exercise promotion and nutritional counseling to improve energy, muscle function, and mood. In children with chronic inflammatory disease, treating underlying inflammation and optimizing vitamin D status may both be needed to achieve symptom relief.

Positioning vitamin D alongside sleep hygiene, nutrition, and psychosocial care allows clinicians to address fatigue as a multidimensional phenomenon rather than a single lab value.

This integrative perspective underscores that managing fatigue requires not just supplementation, but recognition of its biopsychosocial complexity.

Evidence gaps and research priorities

Despite encouraging signals, gaps remain. High-quality, adequately powered pediatric RCTs using validated fatigue instruments, stratified by baseline 25(OH)D, and with standardized dosing regimens are needed. Research should clarify the minimal serum level associated with symptomatic improvement and compare daily versus bolus regimens for fatigue outcomes (López-Muñoz et al., 2023; Filgueiras et al., 2020). Mechanistic studies linking mitochondrial function, inflammatory markers, and objective measures of muscle performance to symptom change will strengthen causal inference. Long-term safety data for higher-dose pediatric regimens used for non-skeletal symptoms remain limited.

Resolving these uncertainties will transform vitamin D from a plausible contributor to a proven lever for improving energy, function, and quality of life in tired children worldwide.

Future scholarship should aim to shift fatigue research from anecdotal associations to reproducible clinical protocols.

Conclusion

Ultimately, the story of fatigue and vitamin D is one of recognition: a common, disruptive symptom linked to a common, correctable deficiency.

Vitamin D deficiency is a biologically plausible and clinically modifiable contributor to fatigue in children. Observational data consistently associate low 25(OH)D with fatigue and related functional impairment, and interventional studies — including recent pediatric trials and systematic reviews — indicate that correction of deficiency can reduce fatigue symptoms in targeted populations. Clinicians evaluating children with unexplained fatigue should consider measuring 25(OH)D when risk factors or refractory symptoms are present and treat confirmed deficiency according to established pediatric protocols, with follow-up to ensure biochemical correction and clinical improvement (Devulapalli et al., 2025; Holick et al., 2011).

Framed this way, vitamin D correction in tired children represents not just nutritional care, but restoration of vigor, growth, and participation in the daily life of childhood.

References

1. Ceglia L. Vitamin D and skeletal muscle tissue and function. Mol Aspects Med. 2009.

2. Di Molfetta IV et al. Vitamin D and fatigue: a narrative review of current evidence. Nutrients. 2024.

3. Dougherty KA et al. Vitamin D supplementation improves quality of life in children with low vitamin D. J Pediatr Health Care. 2020.

4. Devulapalli CS. Vitamin D deficiency and fatigue in children: an overlooked but modifiable factor? World

J Pediatr. Published online September 20, 2025. doi:10.1007/s12519-025-00970-y

5. Filgueiras MS, et al. Vitamin D status, oxidative stress, and inflammation in children and adolescents: A systematic review. Crit Rev Food Sci Nutr. 2020.

6. Finch SL, et al. Vitamin D and juvenile idiopathic arthritis. Pediatr Rheumatol Online J. 2018.

7. Głąbska D, et al. The influence of vitamin D intake and status on mental health in children: a systematic review. Nutrients. 2021.

8. Grudet C et al. Vitamin D and inflammation in major depressive disorder. J Affect Disord. 2020.

9. Högberg G et al. Vitamin D supplementation and mental health outcomes in adolescents. Acta Paediatr. 2012.

10. Holick MF et al. Vitamin D deficiency. N Engl J Med. 2007.

11. Holick MF et al. Evaluation, treatment, and prevention of vitamin D deficiency: Endocrine Society guideline. J Clin Endocrinol Metab. 2011.

12. López-Muñoz P, et al. Effect of Vitamin D Supplementation on Fatigue in Multiple Sclerosis: A

Systematic Review and Meta-Analysis. Nutrients. 2023.

13. Mocayar Marón F, et al. Vitamin D status and fatigue in adolescents. J Pediatr Endocrinol Metab. 2020.

14. Munns CF et al. Global consensus recommendations on prevention and management of nutritional rickets. J Clin Endocrinol Metab. 2016.

15. Nowak A et al. Effect of vitamin D on energy and fatigue: a randomized placebo-controlled trial. Medicine (Baltimore). 2016.

16. Pappa HM, et al. Vitamin D status in children and young adults with inflammatory bowel disease. Pediatrics. 2006.

17. Roy S et al. The role of vitamin D in chronic fatigue and pediatric symptoms. N Am J Med Sci. 2014.

18. Sinha A et al. Effect of vitamin D supplementation on muscle strength and energy metabolism in children. J Clin Endocrinol Metab. 2013.

19. Vehapoglu A et al. Effect of vitamin D supplementation in children with growing pains. Med Princ Pract. 2015.

20. Zhang X et al. Vitamin D deficiency and physical activity in schoolchildren: a cross-sectional study. BMC Pediatr. 2020.

Part IV – Clinical Strategies and Future Horizons

13. Advancing Vitamin D Assessment and Personalized Supplementation Practices in Childhood

Introduction

Vitamin D status in children spans a continuum from subclinical insufficiency to overt deficiency and rickets. While rickets represents the extreme, overt end of this spectrum, the far more common challenge in pediatric practice is the detection and management of vitamin D insufficiency, which may compromise bone mineralization and long-term skeletal health without visible skeletal deformities (Munns et al., 2016; Misra et al., 2008).

Recent guidelines from global, European, Nordic, North American, and Asian pediatric societies converge on the principles of risk-based assessment, preventive supplementation, and targeted treatment, though thresholds and dosing regimens vary (Braegger et al., 2013; Saggese et al., 2018; Pludowski et al., 2018). This chapter presents an evidence-based approach starting with insufficiency and progressing to deficiency and rickets, offering clinicians a practical framework for assessment and supplementation.

By tracing the spectrum from subtle insufficiency to overt rickets, we can better understand vitamin D as both an individual clinical concern and a broader marker of equity in child health.

In this way, vitamin D becomes both a clinical biomarker and a public health litmus test, revealing the success or fragility of preventive systems in place.

Table 3: Recommended Daily Vitamin D Intake in Children

Age Group	Recommended Intake (IU/day) *	Notes
0–12 months	400 IU	Breastfed and formula-fed infants
1–18 years	600 IU	May need more in deficiency settings
High-risk groups (dark skin, veiled, preterm, obese)	800–1000 IU	Individualized dosing

*Based on international guidelines (IOM, ESPGHAN, Endocrine Society).

Vitamin D Insufficiency in Childhood

Definition and epidemiology:

Vitamin D insufficiency is commonly defined as serum 25-hydroxyvitamin D [25(OH)D] levels of 30–50 nmol/L, a range associated with impaired calcium absorption and secondary hyperparathyroidism in some children (Holmlund-Suila et al., 2012; Cashman et al., 2019). Prevalence studies

across Europe, North America, and Asia report insufficiency in 30–70% of children and adolescents, even in sunny countries, due to limited outdoor activity, sunscreen use, veiling, and dietary insufficiency (Holmlund-Suila et al., 2016; Wagner et al., 2020; Zhang et al., 2020).
The breadth of this range highlights that insufficiency is less about scarcity of sunshine alone, and more about lifestyle transitions at the ecological and societal level.

Clinical significance:

Although children with insufficiency often appear healthy, studies demonstrate subtle adverse effects on bone mineral density, peak bone mass acquisition, and markers of bone turnover (Wu et al., 2023). Early intervention through supplementation can restore adequate 25(OH)D levels, improve skeletal health, and support broader systemic benefits (Golden & Abrams, 2014; Ma et al., 2021).

These 'silent' effects remind us that children do not need to show bowed legs to carry the hidden burden of suboptimal vitamin D.
Left unrecognized, insufficiency quietly narrows the developmental window for optimal bone and muscle growth, with repercussions in adulthood.

Assessment:

Routine testing in healthy children is not recommended. Targeted measurement is indicated for children with risk factors such as obesity, chronic illness, malabsorption, dark skin, limited sun exposure, or restrictive diets (Braegger et al., 2013; Corsello et al., 2023). Serum 25(OH)D remains the biomarker of choice, ideally measured using standardized LC-MS/MS or validated immunoassays. Interpretation should be informed by calcium, phosphate, ALP, and PTH in children with borderline levels or clinical concerns (Holmlund-Suila et al., 2013; Cashman et al., 2019).

Standardization of assay methods and consideration of seasonal, geographic, and demographic factors enhance the accuracy and clinical relevance of serum 25(OH)D measurements (EFSA, 2016).

Thus, testing becomes less about chasing numbers, and more about tailoring vigilance to those whose biology or context puts them most at risk.
Assessment is therefore not a broad net, but a targeted probe designed to find deficiency where risk converges.

Supplementation strategies:

- Infants (<12 months): 400–800 IU/day (10–20 μg), especially for exclusively breastfed infants (Cashman et al., 2019; Weiler et al., 2024).

- Children and adolescents: 600–1000 IU/day is typically sufficient to correct insufficiency. Obese children may require higher doses due to volumetric dilution.

- Fortified foods: Dairy, cereals, and oils enhance population coverage, particularly where adherence to supplementation is suboptimal (Holmlund-Suila et al., 2016; Cashman et al., 2019).

Adherence challenges require ongoing education and culturally appropriate interventions to ensure effective and safe supplementation across diverse pediatric populations (Aul et al., 2023; Buttriss et al., 2022).

Here, supplementation and fortification serve as quiet public health levers—small daily doses with lasting generational impact.
These small adjustments at the population scale translate into protection at the individual scale, preventing deficiency before symptoms surface.

Monitoring:

After 3–6 months of supplementation, serum 25(OH)D can be rechecked in high-risk children to ensure sufficiency, while avoiding unnecessary testing in low-risk populations (Pludowski et al., 2018).

Vitamin D Deficiency and Rickets

Definition and pathophysiology:

Deficiency is typically defined as serum 25(OH)D <30 nmol/L. When prolonged, it can lead to clinical rickets, characterized by impaired mineralization, skeletal deformities, delayed growth, and biochemical abnormalities (hypocalcemia, elevated ALP, secondary hyperparathyroidism) (Munns et al., 2016; Misra et al., 2008). Children at risk include infants with low sun exposure, children with malabsorption, those with darker skin in high latitudes, and children on restrictive diets (Chakhtoura et al., 2018).

Clinical presentation:

- Early signs: delayed motor milestones, hypotonia, irritability.
- Progressive rickets: bowing of legs, widening of wrists, rachitic rosary, growth retardation.
- Laboratory findings: low 25(OH)D, low-normal calcium, elevated ALP, raised PTH. Radiographs show metaphyseal cupping and fraying in long bones.

Every rachitic rosary on a chest and every bowed tibia in a child speaks to missed opportunities in prevention. Rickets thus remains a visible indictment of system-level failure, starkly signaling where prevention fell short.

Treatment strategies:

- Mild deficiency (25–30 nmol/L): daily supplementation (800–1000 IU) until levels exceed 50 nmol/L, with monitoring of calcium and ALP (Munns et al., 2016).

- Moderate to severe deficiency/rickets: therapeutic high-dose regimens (e.g., oral cholecalciferol 2000 IU/day for infants, 50,000 IU weekly for older children for 6 weeks) followed by maintenance supplementation (400–1000 IU/day). Hypocalcemia should be corrected concurrently (Munns et al., 2016).

- Special populations: malabsorption, obesity, chronic liver or kidney disease may require individualized, monitored higher doses (Corsello et al., 2023).

Therapeutic dosing must be personalized with vigilant monitoring to prevent complications and maximize clinical outcomes, especially in high-risk groups (Bouftas et al., 2024).

Therapeutic dosing is thus less about reversing visible deformity than about restoring a child's trust in their own bones as they grow.
Here, the aim is to rescue not just bone architecture, but the trajectory of growth and resilience across the lifespan.

Monitoring:

Recheck serum 25(OH)D, calcium, phosphate, and ALP 1–3 months after therapy initiation. Radiographs may be repeated after 3 months to confirm healing (Munns et al., 2016).

Integrating Insufficiency and Deficiency Management

Conceptually, insufficiency and deficiency lie along a spectrum. Early detection and correction of insufficiency can prevent progression to rickets. Population-level interventions (fortification, universal infant supplementation) combined with targeted high-risk strategies (screening, therapeutic dosing) form a continuum of care (Pludowski et al., 2018; Saggese et al., 2018).

Seen as a continuum, insufficiency and rickets are not different conditions but different chapters of the same unfinished story—one that prevention can rewrite.

This spectrum underscores the preventive mandate: stop insufficiency early, and rickets need not appear at all.

Enhancing Global Relevance and Policy Appeal

Modern environmental and lifestyle factors amplify vitamin D deficiency globally. Urbanization, indoor lifestyles, air pollution, and clothing practices reduce safe sunlight exposure even in sunny regions. Seasonal extremes and geographic variation further complicate vitamin D sufficiency, highlighting the need for locally adapted strategies (Cashman et al., 2019; Zhang et al., 2020).

Framing vitamin D programs in terms of health system impact and economics strengthens policy relevance. Investments in supplementation, fortification, and education prevent rickets and deficiency, improve growth and cognitive outcomes, reduce long-term healthcare costs, and mitigate chronic disease risk. Highlighting cost-effectiveness and societal benefits can accelerate adoption and ensure sustainable implementation (Corsello et al., 2023; Buttriss et al., 2022).

Framing vitamin D through health systems and economics reveals it as not merely a nutrient intervention, but as an investment in human potential.
At scale, vitamin D policy represents an equity tool: small doses that help bridge gaps between different socioeconomic and cultural groups worldwide.

Conclusion

In the end, the challenge is not simply detecting deficiency, but building sustainable systems where no child anywhere slips silently from insufficiency into preventable disease.

Vitamin D status in children is a continuum from subclinical insufficiency to overt rickets. Management must prioritize prevention, with universal infant supplementation and targeted dosing in older children, while ensuring that children with insufficiency or deficiency receive evidence-based supplementation. Early recognition, risk-based assessment, and culturally sensitive, region-specific dosing strategies optimize skeletal health and reduce the burden of rickets worldwide (Munns et al., 2016; Misra et al., 2008; Pludowski et al., 2018).

In sum, applying precision supplementation and preventive public health policies can transform vitamin D from a measure of inequity into a guarantee of growth, resilience, and long-term child health.

References

1. Abrams SA, et al. Optimizing bone health in children and adolescents. Pediatrics. 2014.

2. Absoud M, et al. Prevalence and predictors of vitamin D insufficiency in children: a Great Britain population-based study. PLoS One. 2011.

3. Aul AJ, et al. Infant and Maternal Vitamin D Supplementation: Clinician Perspectives and Practices. J Am Board Fam Med. 2023.

4. Bouftas F, et al. Vitamin D and pediatric bone health: Important information and considerations for the pediatric orthopaedic surgeon. Journal of the Pediatric Orthopaedic Society of North America. 2024.

5. Braegger C, et al. Vitamin D in the healthy European paediatric population. J Pediatr Gastroenterol Nutr. 2013.

6. Buttriss JL, et al. Implementation strategies for improving vitamin D status and increasing vitamin D

intake in the UK: current controversies and future perspectives. Br J Nutr. 2022.

7. Cashman KD, et al. Food fortification improves vitamin D status in children: evidence from Nordic countries. Am J Clin Nutr. 2019.

8. Chakhtoura M, et al. Vitamin D in the Middle East and North Africa. Bone Rep. 2018.

9. Corsello A, et al. Vitamin D in pediatric age: Current evidence, recommendations, and misunderstandings. Front Med (Lausanne). 2023.

10. EFSA. Scientific opinion on dietary reference values for vitamin D. EFSA J. 2016.

11. Golden NH, Abrams SA; Committee on Nutrition. Optimizing bone health in children and adolescents. Pediatrics. 2014.

12. Holmlund-Suila E, et al. High-dose vitamin D intervention in infants—effects on vitamin D status, calcium homeostasis, and bone strength. J Clin Endocrinol Metab. 2012.

13. Holmlund-Suila E, et al. Vitamin D deficiency in children with a chronic illness—seasonal and age-related variations in serum 25-hydroxy Vitamin D concentrations. PLoS One. 2013.

14. Kumar J, et al. Prevalence and associations of 25-hydroxyvitamin D deficiency in US children: NHANES 2001-2004. Pediatrics. 2009.

15. Ma K, et al. Effect of vitamin D supplementation in early life on children's growth and body composition: A systematic review and meta-analysis. Nutrients. 2021.

16. Meltzer HM, et al. Challenges and opportunities when moving food production and consumption toward sustainable diets in the Nordics: a scoping review. Food & Nutrition Research. 2023.

17. Misra M, et al. Vitamin D deficiency in children and its management: review of current knowledge and recommendations. Pediatrics. 2008.

18. Munns CF, et al. Global consensus recommendations on prevention and management of nutritional rickets. J Clin Endocrinol Metab. 2016.

19. Mutlu GY, et al. Use of vitamin D in children and adults: frequently asked questions. J Clin Res Pediatr Endocrinol. 2018.

20. Pludowski P, et al. Vitamin D supplementation guidelines. J Steroid Biochem Mol Biol. 2018.

21. Saggese G, et al. Vitamin D in childhood and adolescence: Italian consensus guidelines. Ital J Pediatr. 2018.

22. Weiler HA, et al. Adherence to vitamin D supplementation recommendations for breastfed infants and young children. J Nutr. 2024.

23. Wu F, et al. Vitamin D supplementation for improving bone density in vitamin D-deficient children and adolescents: systematic review and meta-analysis. Am J Clin Nutr. 2023.

24. Zhang H, et al. Status and influential factors of vitamin D among children aged 0 to 6 years in a Chinese population. BMC Public Health. 2020.

14. Synthesizing Evidence in Pediatric Vitamin D Medicine

Introduction

Vitamin D research in pediatrics has entered a new era. Once regarded almost exclusively in relation to rickets, vitamin D is now considered a broader determinant of child health, with implications extending to growth, immunity, and chronic disease risk. This chapter integrates the evidence reviewed in earlier sections of this book, identifies clinical and scientific gaps, and highlights research priorities for the next decade. While the science of vitamin D is well established in its relation to skeletal health, uncertainties remain regarding definitions of insufficiency, the management of suboptimal levels, and the wider relevance of supplementation strategies in diverse pediatric populations.

In bringing these strands together, vitamin D becomes more than a nutrient — it symbolizes the unfinished transition from science to equity in global child health.
Framed this way, vitamin D acts not just as a scientific subject but as a mirror for how societies transform knowledge into practical health equity for children.

Established Knowledge: From Rickets Prevention to Policy Translation

There is little dispute that adequate vitamin D prevents nutritional rickets, and that supplementation in infancy is an essential preventive measure. Global consensus statements confirm that rickets is both preventable and treatable, provided supplementation and fortification policies are in place and adhered to (Munns et al., 2016). Countries such as Finland, which implemented food fortification alongside infant supplementation, have achieved significant improvements in pediatric vitamin D status (Raulio et al., 2017). Similar progress has been documented in Ireland, Canada, and Northern Europe (Cashman et al., 2019).

These successes illustrate that science can directly translate into public health policy. Yet they also highlight persistent inequities: rickets remains present in regions of Africa, South Asia, and the Middle East where supplementation programs are fragmented or absent. Such inequities underscore the importance of implementation science and the need for vitamin D policies that are adapted to local sociocultural and economic realities.

Continued investment in fortification and supplementation programs remains essential to sustain and expand these public health gains globally.

These public health victories remind us that prevention is possible, yet also that its reach is bounded by equity: where systems invest, children thrive; where they do not, rickets still emerges.
Thus, the story of rickets demonstrates both the triumph of applied science and the unfinished duty of global health translation.

The Uncertain Terrain of Vitamin D Insufficiency

In contrast to deficiency and rickets, vitamin D insufficiency represents a less well-defined challenge. Suboptimal levels are associated with potential risks for respiratory infections, asthma, obesity, and immune-mediated disorders, but trial evidence remains inconsistent and often underpowered (Wagner et al., 2008; Golden & Abrams, 2014; Bouftas et al., 2024). This has created uncertainty for clinicians: how aggressively should insufficiency be treated, and at what threshold?

Different guidelines offer varying definitions. ESPGHAN and the American Academy of Pediatrics define sufficiency at ≥50 nmol/L, while other bodies such as the Endocrine Society argue for higher thresholds (Braegger et al., 2013; Misra et al., 2008). The European Food Safety Authority has also issued dietary reference values, adding further complexity (EFSA, 2016). Such variation hampers harmonization of clinical practice and creates confusion among practitioners. Resolving these inconsistencies is a pressing priority for research and consensus-building.

Amidst this uncertainty lies the clinician's dilemma: to treat or to wait, to trust thresholds or to trust trajectories.
Until consensus emerges, clinicians must blend guideline-driven targets with clinical judgment, ensuring no child is left at risk because of arbitrary definitional divides.

Global Health Dimensions and the Role of the United Nations

Beyond the clinic, vitamin D deficiency and insufficiency are deeply embedded in global health inequities. The paradox of deficiency in sun-rich countries points to the importance of sociocultural practices, skin pigmentation, diet, and poverty in shaping children's exposure and access to vitamin D. Many of the most affected populations are also those least studied in large clinical trials, limiting the global applicability of existing evidence.

Furthermore, modern environmental and lifestyle factors amplify deficiency risks worldwide. Urbanization, increased indoor living, air pollution, and changing clothing practices reduce safe sunlight exposure even in sun-rich regions. Coupled with climate variability and seasonal extremes, these factors highlight that vitamin D insufficiency is a dynamic, context-dependent challenge requiring locally adapted strategies.

International agencies such as UNICEF and WHO have long recognized the burden of micronutrient deficiencies as barriers to child health and development. Both organizations emphasize vitamin D within broader strategies for child nutrition, reflected in the UNICEF Global Micronutrient Strategy 2020–2030 and the WHO Micronutrient Action Plan 2021–2030 (UNICEF, 2020; WHO, 2021). These frameworks are directly aligned with the United Nations Sustainable Development Goals, which prioritize reductions in child morbidity and mortality. Yet implementation remains uneven, and vitamin D is often overshadowed by higher-profile micronutrients such as iron or vitamin A. A stronger role for the UN in advocacy, funding, and policy harmonization could reduce the persistent inequities in global vitamin D status among children.

In addition, framing vitamin D programs in economic and health system terms strengthens their appeal to policy makers. Investments in supplementation, fortification, and population education not only prevent rickets and bone deformities but also reduce long-term healthcare costs, improve growth and cognitive outcomes, and mitigate chronic disease risks. Articulating the cost-effectiveness and broader societal benefits of these interventions can accelerate policy adoption and ensure sustainable implementation.

Strengthened advocacy and funding, tailored to regional sociocultural contexts, are critical to address endemic vitamin D deficiencies and promote equity in child health outcomes.

Seen globally, vitamin D is not just about biology, but about justice — a measure of whether children born under different skies are granted the same chance at healthy growth.

Here, vitamin D becomes a barometer of fairness, capturing in a single biomarker the success—or neglect—of public health systems.

Future Research Horizons

Moving forward, three research priorities stand out. First, a harmonized definition of insufficiency and deficiency is required, ideally based on clinical outcomes rather than biochemical thresholds alone (Zhu et al., 2025; StatPearls, 2025). Second, high-risk pediatric groups — including preterm infants, children with chronic diseases, and those with obesity — need targeted studies to determine appropriate supplementation strategies (Bhalla et al., 2025; Mutlu et al., 2018; Frontiers Endocrinology, 2025). Third, the scalability of interventions must be tested in diverse settings. Fortification, supplementation, and school-based health programs offer promising models, but their effectiveness depends on cultural acceptability, political commitment, and economic feasibility (Meltzer et al., 2023; Anales de Pediatría, 2025). Comparative research across different health systems would help establish best practices (Pludowski et al., 2018; Zhu et al., 2025).

Comprehensive, culturally sensitive approaches that bridge basic science, clinical medicine, and public health policy will be pivotal for sustained progress (International Journal of Public Health, 2025; StatPearls, 2025).

The task ahead is to transform scattered insights into common ground, so that research no longer stops at national borders but speaks with a united scientific voice.

To achieve this, pediatric vitamin D science must evolve into a collaborative platform—one that unites researchers, clinicians, and policymakers in the service of shared child health goals.

Conclusion

The journey of vitamin D in pediatrics is both a triumph and a reminder — triumph in the bones made straight where deficiency was corrected, reminder in the millions of children still waiting for those benefits.

Vitamin D in childhood medicine represents a story of both success and unfinished business. The eradication of rickets in many countries demonstrates the power of supplementation and fortification policies, yet the persistence of deficiency and insufficiency elsewhere underscores the challenges of equity, consistency, and translation. Research must now move beyond skeletal endpoints, focus on vulnerable populations, and test scalable interventions across diverse regions. Achieving this will require coordinated action not only from clinicians and researchers but also from governments and international agencies such as the UN. The science is clear; the challenge now is to ensure that every child, regardless of geography or circumstance, can benefit from it.

Ultimately, the legacy of vitamin D in pediatrics will be measured not only in straightened bones, but in whether societies choose to meaningfully close the gaps between knowledge and action.

References

1. Abrams SA, Golden NH; Committee on Nutrition (AAP). Optimizing bone health in children and adolescents. Pediatrics. 2014.

2. Anales de Pediatría. Vitamin D supplementation in the healthy pediatric population: updated clinical recommendations. 2025.

3. Bhalla V, et al. Monitored vitamin D supplementation in preterm infants improves serum status and bone health. Front. Endocrinol. 2025.

4. Bouftas F, et al. Vitamin D and pediatric bone health: Important information and considerations for the pediatric orthopaedic surgeon. Journal of the Pediatric Orthopaedic Society of North America. 2024.

5. Braegger C, et al. ESPGHAN Committee on Nutrition. Vitamin D in the healthy European paediatric population. J Pediatr Gastroenterol Nutr. 2013.

6. Cashman KD, et al. Food fortification improves vitamin D status in children: evidence from Nordic countries. Am J Clin Nutr. 2019.

7. EFSA. Scientific opinion on dietary reference values for vitamin D. EFSA J. 2016.

8. International Journal of Public Health. Vitamin D Deficiency and Associated Factors in Children: A Multicenter Study. 2025.

9. Meltzer HM, et al. Challenges and opportunities when moving food production and consumption toward sustainable diets in the Nordics: a scoping review for Nordic Nutrition Recommendations 2023. Food & Nutrition Research. 2023.

10. Misra M, et al. Drug and Therapeutics Committee of the Lawson Wilkins Pediatric Endocrine Society. Vitamin D deficiency in children and its management: review of current knowledge and recommendations. Pediatrics. 2008.

11. Munns CF, et al. Global consensus recommendations on prevention and management of nutritional rickets. J Clin Endocrinol Metab. 2016.

12. Mutlu GY, et al. Use of vitamin D in children and adults: frequently asked questions. J Clin Res Pediatr Endocrinol. 2018.

13. Pludowski P, et al. Vitamin D supplementation guidelines. J Steroid Biochem Mol Biol. 2018.

14. Raulio S, et al. Successful nutrition policy: improvement of vitamin D intake and status in Finnish adults over the last decade. Eur J Public Health. 2017.

15. StatPearls. Vitamin D Deficiency. National Library of Medicine. 2025.

16. UNICEF. Global Micronutrient Strategy 2020–2030. United Nations Children's Fund; 2020.

17. Wagner CL, Greer FR; American Academy of Pediatrics Section on Breastfeeding; American Academy of Pediatrics Committee on Nutrition. Prevention of rickets and vitamin D deficiency in infants, children, and adolescents. Pediatrics. 2008.

18. WHO. Nutrition for Health and Development: Micronutrient Action Plan 2021–2030. World Health Organization; 2021.

19. Zhu Q, et al. Different diagnostic criteria influence the determination of Vitamin D nutritional status in children: a cross-sectional study. Front. Public Health. 2025.

Concluding Synthesis: Vitamin D in Childhood Health and Equity

From Bones to Systems: Expanding the Narrative of Vitamin D

Across the 14 chapters of this book, vitamin D has been followed from the narrow, skeletal lens of rickets prevention to its wider roles in immunity, growth, neurodevelopment, and chronic disease vulnerability. The classical story—sunlight, diet, bone strength—remains foundational, yet modern research shows vitamin D acting across multiple biological systems, linking nutrition and lifestyle to immunity, fatigue, obesity, and allergic and respiratory conditions.

A central theme that emerges is interconnectedness: vitamin D status is not determined by a single risk factor but by the interplay of sunlight, culture, body composition, immune function, genetics, and socioeconomic environment. Deficiency, therefore, becomes not merely the absence of a micronutrient but the visible endpoint of wider ecological, sociocultural, and systemic forces surrounding childhood.

Clinical Themes: Detection, Diagnosis, and Management

1. **Spectrum Thinking:** Chapters 1, 2, and 13 established vitamin D status as a continuum from insufficiency to deficiency to overt rickets. Children

may appear clinically well while accruing silent disadvantages in bone density, peak growth, and fatigue. Clinical practice, therefore, requires vigilance in recognizing insufficiency before it progresses to visible disease.

2. Targeted Assessment: Recurrent across chapters is the consensus that testing should be selective and risk-based—not routine but guided by circumstances such as obesity, chronic disease, darker skin pigmentation, or limited sun exposure (Ch. 3, 7, 12, 13).

3. Personalized Supplementation: Multiple chapters—on obesity, fatigue, and insufficiency—converge on one lesson: "one-size-fits-all" supplementation is inadequate. Body mass index, inflammatory states, cultural practices, and genetic polymorphisms must inform dosing. Personalized regimens, aligned with monitoring, form the new horizon of pediatric supplementation.

4. Integration with Broader Care: Vitamin D is best addressed not in isolation but as part of a holistic evaluation that considers sleep, nutrition, physical activity, inflammatory status, and psychosocial context (Ch. 6, 8, 12).

Scientific Insights Beyond Bone Health

- **Immune Modulation:** Evidence from asthma (Ch. 9), RTIs (Ch. 10), and autoimmune conditions (Ch. 8) demonstrates vitamin D's active role in immune regulation—amplifying innate defenses, tempering excess inflammation, and possibly modulating disease activity.

- **Neuro-muscular and Fatigue Pathways:** Chapters 6 and 12 highlighted mechanisms through which vitamin D modulates muscle strength and oxidative metabolism, linking deficiency to fatigue—a subtle but functionally disruptive pediatric symptom.

- **Allergic and Atopic Disease:** Chapters 9 and 11 underscored vitamin D's involvement in Th2/Th1 balance, barrier integrity, and atopic manifestations, positioning it as a potential modifier of the "atopic march."

- **Obesity and Functional Deficiency:** Chapter 7 reframed deficiency in obese children as a functional deficit—due not to intake, but to sequestration, metabolic dysregulation, and inflammatory signaling.

These themes collectively argue that vitamin D is not only a skeletal guardian but also an integrated regulator of growth, energy, and immune resilience.

Public Health Dimensions and Global Equity

Chapters 3, 4, and 5 placed vitamin D within the broad contours of population health. Deficiency persists paradoxically in sun-rich regions, reaffirming that sunlight abundance does not automatically equate to sufficiency. Air pollution, cultural practices, migration, urbanization, and health system gaps are the true determinants—reminders that deficiency is as much a marker of inequity as of biology.

- **North–South paradox:** Rickets in sunny countries (Ch. 5) reveals system-level failures in supplementation, fortification, and maternal-child services.

- **Global Diversity:** Immigrant children in northern latitudes (Ch. 3) exemplify how cultural identity, pigmentation, and policy intersect to shape vulnerability.

- **Policy Levers:** The strongest success stories—Finland, Canada, Nordic countries (Ch. 14)—demonstrated that sustained fortification plus universal supplementation reliably prevent rickets and reduce insufficiency.

Thus, vitamin D becomes a policy-sensitive nutrient, one whose sufficiency (or lack thereof) reflects broader investments in prevention and equity.

Persistent Gaps and Research Priorities

Building on Chapter 14's synthesis, several research frontiers remain urgent:

- Defining harmonized thresholds of sufficiency based on outcomes beyond skeletal health.
- Understanding optimal supplementation in high-risk groups: preterm infants, obese children, and those with inflammatory conditions.
- Long-term, multicenter trials testing integrated interventions (supplementation plus fortification plus education) across diverse cultural and health system contexts.
- Mechanistic studies clarifying mitochondrial, immune, and microbiome pathways linking vitamin D to fatigue, infection, and allergy.

The central methodological challenge is precision: tailoring definitions, monitoring, and interventions in ways that respect biological diversity and social context.

Broader Reflection: Vitamin D as a Measure of Childhood Health and Justice

Stepping back, the threads woven across these chapters present vitamin D as both molecule and metaphor. It is a molecule essential for growth, bone integrity, immunity, and energy. But it is also a metaphor for how childhood health cannot be separated from context: housing, diet, air, skin, migration, poverty, and policy all converge to determine whether a child is deficient or sufficient.

Philosophically, vitamin D teaches us that health is not simply inherited through biology or climate, but actively mediated by culture, equity, and systems of care.

In a 21st-century world marked by paradoxes—sunlight yet rickets, guidelines yet gaps, science yet inequity—ensuring vitamin D sufficiency becomes almost a justice project, a small but concrete guarantee of childhood resilience. To correct deficiency is to correct not merely a biochemical imbalance, but a systemic one: the right of every child, regardless of geography or circumstance, to grow with strength, vitality, and equal opportunity for health.

Epilogue

Illuminating the Path from Molecule to Meaning — The Promise of Vitamin D in Childhood

As this volume draws to a close, the journey of vitamin D—from its molecular dance in cells to its profound imprint on the lives of children worldwide—resonates as a parable of science in service to humanity. What began as a story of preventing rachitic bows and brittle bones has evolved into a saga of nurturing resilience: of building immune defenses, nurturing growth, lifting fatigue, and tempering the storms of allergy and infection.

This narrative is not merely about a nutrient, but about the orchestration of biology and environment, culture and policy, knowledge and action. Vitamin D emerges as both a guardian molecule and a measuring stick—reflecting how well societies marshal resources, knowledge, and will to protect their youngest citizens.

Yet amid progress, the unfinished chapters of this story remain poignant. Sunlit skies do not guarantee sufficiency. The shadows of inequity—shaped by poverty, migration, urbanization, and climate—still obscure access to this simple protection for millions. Our scientific understanding calls upon us not only to polish assays and perfect dosing regimens but to amplify the voices of those unheard, to reform policies entrenched in disparity, and to craft health systems rooted in justice.

In this light, vitamin D transcends biochemistry to become an emblem of childhood's fundamental promise: that all children deserve the chance to rise to their full potential, with strong bones, vigorous immunity, clear minds, and joyful days.

As researchers and clinicians, scholars and policy-makers, we hold a shared mandate: to close the gap between what we know and what children experience; to translate molecular insights into global health gains; and to ensure that the gift of sunlight's vitamin reaches every child, no matter where they are born.

May this book serve not only as a repository of knowledge but as a beacon guiding that journey—from molecules illuminated in the lab, to lives illuminated with health and hope.

Appendix - Abbreviations

$1,25(OH)_2D$ – 1,25-dihydroxyvitamin D (active form)

25(OH)D – 25-hydroxyvitamin D

AAP – American Academy of Pediatrics

AD – Atopic Dermatitis

AI – Adequate Intake

ALP – Alkaline Phosphatase

AR – Allergic Rhinitis

BMI – Body Mass Index

BMI-for-age – Body Mass Index-for-age percentile

BMC – Bone Mineral Content

BMD – Bone Mineral Density

CF – Cystic Fibrosis

COVID-19 – Coronavirus Disease 2019

CRP – C-Reactive Protein

CYP24A1 – 24-hydroxylase enzyme

CYP27B1 – 1-alpha hydroxylase enzyme

DBP – Vitamin D Binding Protein

DXA – Dual-energy X-ray Absorptiometry

EASI – Eczema Area and Severity Index

ELISA – Enzyme-Linked Immunosorbent Assay

ESPGHAN – European Society for Paediatric Gastroenterology, Hepatology and Nutrition

ESR – Erythrocyte Sedimentation Rate

FEF25-75 – Forced Expiratory Flow 25–75%

FEV1 – Forced Expiratory Volume in 1 second

FGF23 – Fibroblast Growth Factor 23

FVC – Forced Vital Capacity

GI – Gastrointestinal

Hb – Hemoglobin

HPLC – High-Performance Liquid Chromatography

HR – Hazard Ratio

Ig – Immunoglobulin

IgA – Immunoglobulin A

IgE – Immunoglobulin E

IgG – Immunoglobulin G

IgM – Immunoglobulin M

IL – Interleukin

IL-1β – Interleukin-1 beta

IL-6 – Interleukin-6

IL-10 – Interleukin-10

IL-17 – Interleukin-17

JIA – Juvenile Idiopathic Arthritis

LC-MS/MS – Liquid Chromatography-Tandem Mass Spectrometry

MCH – Mean Corpuscular Hemoglobin

MCV – Mean Corpuscular Volume

MMP – Matrix Metalloproteinase

MS – Multiple Sclerosis

mRNA – Messenger Ribonucleic Acid

NF-κB – Nuclear Factor Kappa-light-chain-enhancer of activated B cells

NFAT – Nuclear Factor of Activated T-cells

NTD – Neural Tube Defect

OA – Osteoarthritis

OR – Odds Ratio

OTU – Operational Taxonomic Unit

PCR – Polymerase Chain Reaction

PCV – Packed Cell Volume

PTH – Parathyroid Hormone

RCT – Randomized Controlled Trial

RD – Respiratory Distress

ROC – Receiver Operating Characteristic

ROS – Reactive Oxygen Species

RR – Relative Risk

RTI – Respiratory Tract Infection

SCF – Stem Cell Factor

SCORAD – Scoring Atopic Dermatitis

SD – Standard Deviation

SNP – Single Nucleotide Polymorphism

SLE – Systemic Lupus Erythematosus

TNF – Tumor Necrosis Factor

TNF-α – Tumor Necrosis Factor-alpha

Treg – Regulatory T cell

URTI – Upper Respiratory Tract Infection

UVB – Ultraviolet B Radiation

UVR – Ultraviolet Radiation

VDBP – Vitamin D Binding Protein

VDD – Vitamin D Deficiency

VDI – Vitamin D Insufficiency

VDR – Vitamin D Receptor

VD – Vitamin D

WHO – World Health Organization

z-score – Standard Score

Unlocking the Secrets of Vitamin D: A Comprehensive Guide to Pediatric Health

Dr. Chandra Sekhar Devulapalli MD, PhD, a pediatrician with over three decades of clinical and research experience, presents a definitive exploration of vitamin D's vital role in child health. Once primarily associated with bone health and rickets prevention, vitamin D is now recognized as a key factor in immunity, growth, and chronic disease risk among children worldwide.

This authoritative volume traces vitamin D's evolving story—from molecular pathways to community health strategies—through fourteen thoughtful chapters that integrate cutting-edge science, clinical insights, and public health perspectives. Drawing on global case studies spanning diverse populations, Dr. Devulapalli highlights the complexities of assessment, personalized supplementation, and prevention across varied environments and vulnerable groups.

Designed for pediatricians, researchers, and policymakers alike, the book offers a practical framework for diagnosis, management, and policy development—underscoring vitamin D's emerging role in respiratory infections, allergic diseases, fatigue, and beyond. It also charts future research priorities and advocates for coordinated action to close persistent gaps in equity.

Unlock new horizons in pediatric care with Dr. Devulapalli's expert guidance, ensuring every child has the foundation for a healthy, resilient future.

www.ingramcontent.com/pod-product-compliance
Lightning Source LLC
Chambersburg PA
CBHW031324230926
51848CB00001B/87
* 9 7 8 8 2 6 9 4 3 4 4 2 2 *